Paul Leendertse

THE ROOT CAUSE OF CANCER
How to Begin Healing from Within

Paul Leendertse
What's in a Tear — Book 1

THE ROOT
CAUSE
OF CANCER

How to Begin Healing from Within

What's in a Tear – Book 1
The Root Cause of Cancer – How to Begin Healing from Within

Author: Paul Leendertse
Design: Karin Gleichner, k-designstudio.ch
Editor: Deborah Lynn Jones, Ariane Konrad
Illustrator: Andrea Carroll
Proof Reader: Sofiya Chorniy
Original Edition: Copyright © 2012 Canadian Intellectual
Property Office (What's in a Tear – The Purpose of Cancer)

ISBN: 978-0-9918265-0-6

2nd Edition title change: Copyright © 2020 Canadian Intellectual Property Office (What's in a Tear Book 1: The Root Cause
of Cancer – How to Begin Healing from Within)

3rd Edition – 2023

ISBN: 978-0-9918265-1-3

DISCLAIMER

This book is designed to provide information and motivation to the reader. It is sold with the understanding that the author and publisher are not engaged to render any type of psychological, medical, legal or any other kind of professional advice. The content is the sole expression and opinion of its author. No warranties or guarantees are expressed or implied by the writer's/publisher's choice to include any of the content in this volume. While every attempt has been made to provide accurate information, the author and publisher cannot be held responsible for any errors or omissions. The final decision to engage in any medical treatment should be made jointly by you and your doctor. The author and publisher cannot accept any responsibility for any damage or harm caused by any treatment, advice or information contained in this publication.

CONTENTS

THANK YOU   9

ABOUT THE AUTHOR   11

FOREWORD BY PAUL CHEK   14

THE PARADIGM SHIFT   19

1   CANCER IS NOT WHAT WE THINK IT IS   22

2   YOUR BODY DOESN'T LIE   31

3   ENDING THE WAR ON CANCER   38

4   OUR BODY'S SURVIVAL RESPONSES   49

5   MANAGING BLOOD GLUCOSE   59

6   FIGHT OR FLIGHT   66

7   THE SPECIAL ABILITY OF CANCER CELLS   80

8   100 POUNDS OF POISON   92

9   POISON DISGUISED   101

10   FOOD AND "FOOD"   112

11   CHRONIC STRESS CAN TRIGGER CANCER   129

12   CANCERS LOCATION IS NOT RANDOM   145

13   IT'S NOT OUR BODY'S FAULT   157

14   OUR BODIES FACILITATE THE GROWTH OF CANCER CELLS 166

15   YOU CAN PREVENT AND REVERSE CANCER   175

16   THE CURE IS YOU, AND ALL OF US   184

REFERENCES   189

THANK YOU

For several years I have been putting together a puzzle, and each piece, although difference and unique, is essential to the whole.

I have spent a great deal of time learning the various aspects of health – what creates it and sustains it. This includes the workings of the physical body, nutrition, emotional well-being, farming (such as the importance of soil health and its effect on nutrient density of plants), spirituality (for example, how does our beliefs about GOD or SOURCE influence our health? and what is Spirituality anyway?), and much more. I've studied the work of many researchers to aid my discoveries about cancer. Perhaps most valuable, is my extensive work directly with individuals with cancer: by living together with cancer patients for 3 weeks at a time, assessing and investigating every aspect of their lives I could, to understand what caused their cancer. This revealed to me the deeper causes of cancer. Thank you to all the independent thinkers, researchers, authors, and individuals devoted to healing from within, to unravel the truth about cancer.

Thank you to my family and friends. You have not only allowed me to fully express my passions over the years, but provided constructive feedback along the way. Many of you put a lot of time and energy – and your heart – into helping make this book as valuable as it could be. Paul Jackson, Kent Allen, Gavin

Dobias, Steve Assel, Riley McGahey, Michelle Leendertse, my Mother, Rebecca and Susan Hillebrand, Rick and Wendy Jackson, Mike Jackson and many more.

A special thanks to Melissa Falconer and Andrea Carroll for all of your love, energy, and support – you played an essential role in my life, learning invaluable life lessons with me which helped make this book so valuable.

Thank you Aria, for showing up exactly when I needed you most, to refine and "perfectionize" Book 1. I can't ever thank you enough. Your energy and intelligence is within every page of this book. Your beautiful heart is behind so much of my life. You will always be an Angel to me.

Thank you to my stepfather Bill Hooper, and my best friend's father Steve Dobias, who both died of lung cancer; your painful losses in 2008 revealed to me a serious lacking in the understanding of cancer in both the mainstream medical and alternative fields of health.

Thank you Paul Chek. If I hadn't met you back in 2004 and began an intense mentorship with you, I surely would not have developed such a deep understanding of the physical factors, and some of the spiritual factors, related to health and wellbeing. You were a big inspiration on my path.

ABOUT THE AUTHOR

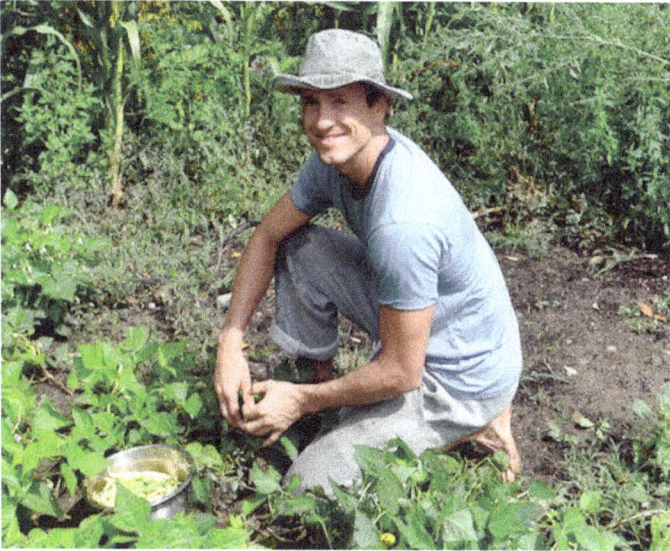

Before authoring the "Root Cause of Cancer" (Book 1 of the *What's in a Tear* Series, first published in 2012), Paul graduated with an Honours Degree in Kinesiology from the University of Waterloo, in Ontario, Canada. After graduating, he then practiced as a CHEK Practitioner and Holistic Lifestyle Coach, trained by the CHEK Institute in California.

When 2 of Pauls family members died of cancer, he began focusing entirely on identifying the Root Cause of Cancer, which launched Paul into a deep journey into the psycho-emotional and spiritual associations with cancer. Paul theorized that cancer must be caused by more than physical factors - stress must be a major component of the cause of cancer.

After he finished his first book, The Root Cause of Cancer, cancer patients who had either stage 3, 4, or "terminal cancer" - most of whom had tried everything to heal - began to seek Pauls help. They had been told nothing more could be done and that they had a limited time to live. However, after reading Paul's book, they knew they had to connect with him, because they realized the stress in their life was connected to their cancer.

This led to Paul's rare opportunity to work one-on-one with Stage 3 and 4 cancer patients for 3 weeks at a time in his "Reverse Cancer Residency", which uncovered rare knowledge of the Root Cause of Cancer. The commitment to self-healing from Pauls clients was invaluable, gradually leading him to developing his 15 Step Self-Healing Process, which he teaches in his Level 1 Root Cause Practitoner Training, followed by his 28 Step Cancer Reversal Process, taught in his advanced Level 2 Training. www.rootcauseinstitute.com

Paul's first client is still cancer-free today, along with many others. Working with Paul, clients have effectively reversed their cancer by identifying the root cause of their particular cancer and what changes they needed to make to reverse it.

Paul's theory that cancer is caused by the accumulation of chronic stress in the body has become a fact – at least for him and his clients, for whom it's become obvious after looking deeper into their personal life challenges associated with their cancer diagnosis. At the time of this writing, 90% of Paul's clients in his residency program have reversed their cancer by devoting themselves to a process of positive life-transformation.

Paul does not heal or cure people – he teaches that the only way a person can heal long term, is through their own self-healing process. Paul's role is to help individuals successfully navigate that process.

FOREWORD BY PAUL CHEK

What's in a Tear – All of you!

Though *What's in a Tear* is a book primarily about cancer, it is essential to realize from the beginning that cancer is a **late stage manifestation of excess stress adaptation**. Prior to the arrival of cancer or any other disease state, there are always a variety of stressors along the way that have not been effectively perceived, or addressed. We know this for sure because disease is not a natural state – health is. Our body and mind naturally seek balance.

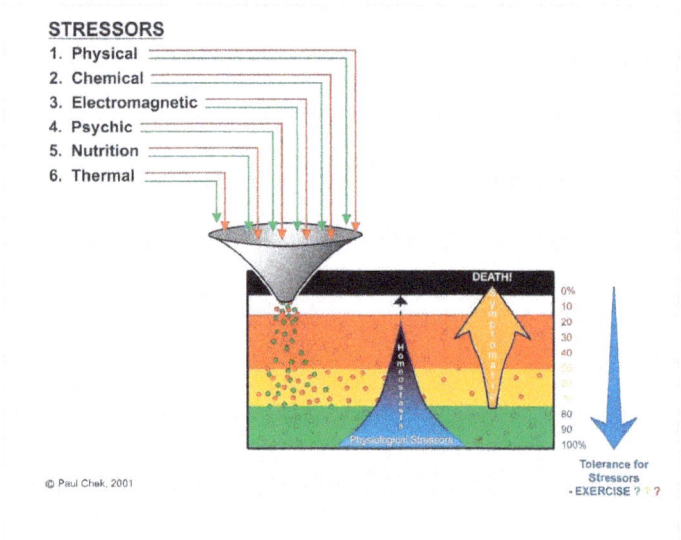

STRESSORS
1. Physical
2. Chemical
3. Electromagnetic
4. Psychic
5. Nutrition
6. Thermal

© Paul Chek, 2001

Tolerance for Stressors
- EXERCISE ? ? ?

Though stress has become a somewhat dirty word, most always implying that something is wrong in our lives, **stress is essential to healthy living.** As you can see in my diagram above, there are six primary stressors to which we all need exposure if we are to grow and flourish effectively as human beings. The green arrows represent healthy doses of each stress type, while the red arrows indicate the potential influence of too much or too little.

What most people fail to realize (medical professionals included), is that **all stressors summate [add up]** within us, to create a "total stress load". When our total stress load is within our capacity to balance, we are in **homeostasis – functional balance;** homeostasis is represented as green in the diagram. In homeostasis, we are able to experience, learn, and grow from our exposure to stressors. In homeostasis, we typically have the reserves of energy and resources to bounce back from stress (allostasis).

A simple example of homeostasis and allostasis can be explained through the use of a hammer. If we are not used to working with a hammer, a day's work with one can cause noticeable discomfort in our arm, shoulder and neck (allostasis); now we are in the yellow zone in the diagram. If we wake up sore from using a hammer the previous day, and do some stretching, get a massage, or take the day off, we can usually return to our project again without pain; we return to homeostasis, or the green zone.

If we ignore the discomfort, or decide we don't have time to care for ourselves, and continue to hammer away in discomfort, stress begins to accumulate in our body-mind systems; we are now in the red zone of my diagram. Each time we do that, it's like taking money out of the bank; if you don't put any back in, you encourage bankruptcy (death), not balance. Eventually, you run out of energy, resources, and ways to compensate. Each step of the way, as our energy levels and resources diminish, **our capacity to make changes, and our willingness to eat supportively, move adequately, and take responsibility for our own well-being diminishes...**

So, what do many people do today? They go to a doctor who gives them a diagnosis (like tendonitis) and pills that are designed to take the pain away. Now, in the absence of pain perception, such people continue swinging their hammer. Sooner than later, the pills are not able to stop the pain and another, yet stronger prescription is given. Meanwhile, more and more energy and resources are consumed to deal with the pain, the compensation, and to detoxify the body of the chemicals in the pills. What started out simply as soreness, now turns into something much more challenging, like a torn rotator cuff, a neck strain, or a pinched nerve; soon an operating table is inevitable!

Paul Leendertse (the author of this book) has been a friend and student of mine through the CHEK Institute for over eighteen years. In that time, I've witnessed his own personal growth and transformation process. He has had to deal with cancer in his family. This topic is very real for him, as I'm sure it is for many of you.

Paul has been lovingly devoted in his search for what causes cancer and disease in general. He has read hundreds of books and research articles in the process, but more importantly, he has deeply immersed himself in the study and practice of holistic health. He is a vibrant, very intelligent man who offers his love and experience to you in this amazing series of books.

Your "What's in a Tear" Series covers every essential aspect of holistic living and how it relates to creating health, or disease. He offers a fresh approach to cancer, suggesting that cancer may well be your body's response to excess body-mind stress. His rationale is sound, based on my own clinical experiences working with a wide variety of cancer patients and diseases in general.

Paul leaves no stone unturned as he guides you through the historical approaches and beliefs about cancer. "What's in a Tear" is a book series that will offer you all the awareness needed to lead you to the tools you need to create a healthy body-mind.

This book series is the product of a long process of study and practice in the field of holistic health. Paul is a well-trained and skilled Holistic Lifestyle Coach. He has significant first-hand experience with the power of effective self-management and the use of natural remedies as a prerequisite to invasive approaches to disease.

When you study "What's in a Tear" you will come to realize that the cure for cancer and other disease has been here all along – it is you, provided you understand what it takes to maintain a healthy body-mind and immune system.

Once a person has a deep understanding of body-mind health, they at once understand the absolute importance of caring for our planet with equal love and respect. Our air, food, and water all represent the outside world entering our inner-world of self. If you could take a magic pill that would clean and tune you within, the effects would be lost as soon as you walked into any room built of commercial, toxic materials. It would also disappear as soon as you stepped out the door into the environment so common in most cities and rural (commercial) farming areas today.

The factory that makes the "perfect cancer/disease pill" will most likely be one of the major contributors to the very cause the pill attempts to address, creating a self-defeating prophecy.

Paul Leendertse is among a very small minority of health pioneers who have devoted their lives to telling you the whole truth about cancer, and disease in general. Like any good practitioner of holistic health, he doesn't just burden you will gloom and doom, **he offers a wide variety of viable, available solutions that anyone can use to live a full life, free of disease.** I can't recommend "What's in a Tear" enough.

The "What's in a Tear" Series is an incredible source of knowledge for creating a high degree of health and happiness in one's life. No matter how challenged you may feel about your health right now, know that you have found the book(s) to which your soul was so graciously guiding you. Simply read as much as you can practically apply each day or week. Each day of living holistically, you will be creating health.

Disease cannot exist in the presence of health! If treating diseases has not worked for you, I assure you, creating health and well-being will.

Love and Chi,

Paul Chek
Founder, C.H.E.K. Institute

THE PARADIGM SHIFT

Before you learn what cancer really is, what causes it, and how to prevent and reverse it, I need to make sure you really want to know the truth. "Why would I not?", you may ask. The reason is that, sometimes, the truth can be extremely challenging or painful to accept. Additionally, the truth comes with responsibility, and if you're not ready to take serious responsibility for your own life and your contribution to the world at large, the new awareness you will gain may only feel like a burden.

Book 1 is primarily focused on the effects of physical, mental, and emotional stress on our physiology which may contribute to the development of cancer. Book 2 focuses strictly on the psycho-emotional causes of cancer. Lastly, Book 3 will delve deeply into the Spiritual Causes of cancer, and how and why society needs to change to truly resolve cancer.

Our world needs to change, dramatically (we have huge problems in many realms of life). Our planet has become more and more polluted; our soils, water and air have become largely contaminated with microplastics, pesticides, and other corporate-made contaminants. Forests and wildlife are disappearing. Many families are broken: marriages hardly last anymore, and if they do they're often dealing with an assortment of stressful challenges, that remain unresolved. Childhood cancer is becoming normalized, the incidence of cancer overall is 1 in

2 people[1], and heart disease is the leading cause of death in many "advanced" countries such as the United States[2]. Need I say more to motivate you to contribute to a new reality? This book series is going to provide many solutions for those who are ready to engage in the healing process of change.

Merriam-Webster Dictionary defines a paradigm shift as "an important change that happens when the usual way of thinking about, or doing something, is replaced by a new and different way". Reversing cancer and eventually ending it, requires exactly this – a paradigm shift.

The longstanding paradigm of cancer has been the "War on Cancer". I invite you to begin the process of learning how to heal from within, thereby contributing to a new paradigm, and the end of cancer. Rather than focusing on eliminating cancer, this book will help you focus on eliminating/healing the cause of the cancer.

> *To end cancer, we must stop the war mentality, and instead learn how to heal from within.*

CHANTAL'S CANCER REVERSAL

I had been diagnosed with breast cancer in 2008. I had no family history of cancer, did not take the contraceptive pill, breastfed my 3 children, was physically active and ate a balanced organic diet. This cancer made no sense to me.

My treatment process included a lumpectomy and then 3 months later, a revised margin lumpectomy. I was told that in my case, radiation may or may not help, so I chose to forgo it. Three and a half years later my cancer returned at a rate that justified a double mastectomy. When I went back to see my oncological surgeon, she was upset to tell me that they had not been able to remove all of the cancer. I was against radiation and chemotherapy, however, under advisement from my specialists, I went through 25 treatments in 5 weeks and took Tamoxifen for 2 months. These treatments were never solving my number one priority: the cause of my cancer.

After reading The Root Cause of Cancer, my cancer finally made sense to me… I went to Wheel of Life's 3-Week Reverse Cancer Program and it was a revelation for me. Through life coaching, self-exploration, meditation, a calm place to be, connection to nature, play and good fun, I felt revived. This place was an oasis of wholeness and goodness. Paul helped me see my life and the events in it that shaped me mentally and emotionally. He also helped me believe that I was the only one who could make the required changes in my life to be healed permanently, and he gave me specific direction for those changes.

When I went back home, I kept up with my meditation and used the strategies he taught me to deal with my emotional triggers. I feel empowered, happy, alive, and most of all, I am cancer-free. I realize now that my cancer helped me grow into a stronger, happier person, and now I can be grateful for it.

1

CANCER IS NOT WHAT WE THINK IT IS

For over a hundred years people have been trying to cure cancer with the same general approach (destroy cancer), yet there is still no medical cure – only an ongoing attempt to increase "survival time". [3] As many people have experienced - either directly, or through affected friends or family members - individuals who develop cancer and destroy it using the standard medical approach often have had their cancer re-grow; usually leading to a tragic end of the individual's life.

Current, traditional attempts to solve the world's cancer problem are based on a *theory* about cancer – is this theory really serving us? Theories can be accepted and considered fact for decades, yet dropped entirely when new, relevant information is discovered. Progress has occurred in this way throughout history.

Cancer is not new; the first writings about cancer date back to at least 3000 BCE. [4]

In 400 BCE, Hippocrates (universally recognized as the father of modern medicine) believed that the body had four 'humours' (fluids affecting our physiology): blood, phlegm, yellow and black bile. When the humours were balanced, a person was healthy, but too much or too little of any of the humours caused disease. An excess of black bile in various parts of the body was thought to cause cancer. This theory was embraced and incorporated into the medical teachings of others, and continued through the Middle Ages for over 1300 years.[5]

In the 1600s, the contagion theory of cancer was publicized by Lusitani and Tulp, based on their experience with breast cancer in members of the same household. They proposed that cancer patients should be isolated, preferably outside of cities and towns, to prevent the spread of cancer. The very first hospital built in France was forced to move from the city because people feared cancer would spread.[6]

Around 150 years later in 1761, the first use of autopsies occurred, in an attempt to relate a patient's illness to pathological findings after death. This laid the foundation of oncology – the study of cancer.[7]

In the 1700s, Stahl and Hoffman theorized that cancer was composed of fermenting and degenerating lymph. The lymph theory gained rapid support, and John Hunter, a Scottish surgeon from the 1700s, agreed that tumours grew from lymph constantly excreted by the blood.[8]

In the late 1700s, John Hunter suggested that some cancers might be cured by surgery, but after routine surgery began, cancer was found to grow back, which is still common today and well-documented in the medical community.[9]

Cancer recurrence after surgery led Professor Rudolf Virchow to declare: "The body is a cell state in which every cell is a citizen. Disease is merely the conflict of the citizens of the state brought about by the action of external forces." Virchow also disagreed with Pasteur's germ theory of disease at the time, proposing instead that, "Germs seek their natural habitat – diseased tissue – rather than being the cause of diseased tissue." He thought social factors, such as poverty, were the major cause of diseases, and the way to combat epidemics was political not medical. **His proposal was that the cause of cancer was chronic irritation.**[10]

From the late 1800s until the 1920s, trauma was then thought to be the cause of cancer and was partially supported by experimental studies in mice, where repetitive wounding induced tumours.[11]

As you will learn in the "What's in a Tear" Series, both trauma and chronic irritation are indeed very much in alignment with my observations in my clinical practice as a Root Cause Practitioner. Yet, these theories were unfortunately abandoned before they were fully understood.

In the 1800s, anesthesia was developed which enabled surgery to flourish and the radical mastectomy (breast removal) began as an attempt to cure cancer, **despite prior discoveries in the 1700s which showed cancer grew back after surgery.**[12]

In the late 1900s, a new cancer theory developed which said damage to DNA by chemicals, radiation, viruses, or inherited defective genes, caused normal cells to mutate into cancer cells.[13]

Further research into DNA and genetics led to today's mainstream accepted theory about cancer – that specific genetic errors are the cause of cancer. The idea is that when a set of genes (termed oncogenes) are damaged, it causes normal cells to mutate. Normally, mutated cells are identified by our body and told to self-destruct (apoptosis). However, in the context of cancer, there's a malfunction in tumour suppressor genes, which are responsible for regulating cell division, repairing DNA errors, and initiating cell death. These malfunctions contribute to the emergence and proliferation of cancer cells.[14]

However, more recent research carried out by the MD Anderson Cancer Center, shows that **oncogenes are not the cause of cancer:** "Oncogene activation appears not only in cancer **but also in normal physiology and non-cancer pathology processes".**[15]

Back in 1971, United States President Richard Nixon officially declared "the War on Cancer": a vow that cancer would be cured by 1976.[16] Now, five decades later, we are still at war with cancer – a focus on attacking and destroying cancer cells.

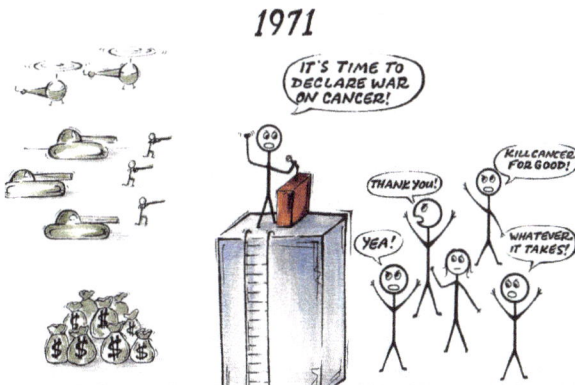

1971

We know that the reality of cancer has been worsening: The chances of developing cancer in 1900 were only 1 in 30.[17] Today, cancer is the highest cause of death in Canada – more than any other source, including heart disease and accidents.[18] Based on 2015 statistics by the Canadian Cancer Society, **1 in 2 Canadians are diagnosed with cancer in their lifetime, and half of them die within 5 years, despite treatments.**[19] About 600,000 Americans are expected to die of cancer in 2020, which translates to about 1600 deaths per day – cancer is the second most common cause of death in the US, exceeded only by cardiovascular disease.[20] According to Britain's 2020 cancer statistics, each year there are 400,000 cases of cancer and 50% of those diagnosed die, despite treatments.[21] Globally, cancer is responsible for about 26,000 deaths per day.[22]

During the last 100 years or so, the mainstream accepted theory of cancer being the result of an error made by our body, and the primary focus of treatment has been on destroying cancer. Simultaneously, cancer incidence and mortality has become so common that the average individual knows at least one friend, colleague, or family member who has died of cancer.

Today, doctors wouldn't be caught dead recommending their patients take up smoking, yet, consider the following advertisement for cigarettes from just a few decades ago. Thus, it is always important that we remember to think for ourselves, so that we can change when change is needed; as has been the case for many patients who have needed to take matters into their own hands when the mainstream medical system has told them nothing could be done, or provided a diagnosis they sensed was inaccurate.

Almost everyone in society has come to believe that the appearance of cancer cells in an individual's body serves no purpose, and its development is largely out of their control. Cancer is often referred to as some kind of aggressive, malignant and rather predatory cell that can strike anyone at any time, for almost no apparent reason. After all, cancer's just a mutated cell that multiplies out of control – right?

Yet, there are cases reported in which a person's cancer mysteriously disappears without any intervention other than making personal life-changes.[24] What exactly did they change? How could the cancer have disappeared if it was indeed a cell that always multiplies out of control? People can live with their cancer in remission (it doesn't grow back after being destroyed) for years beyond their statistically-based prognosis, after choosing to forgo further traditional treatment protocols.[25] Cures that involved no attempt to destroy cancer cells have been labeled "spontaneous remissions" which essentially means, "We don't know why this person's cancer went away – it must be an anomaly" (just like the development of cancer itself: a random cellular mistake.)

In Book 1, *The Root Cause of Cancer*, we will begin exploring an entirely new possibility of what cancer is and what causes it – a paradigm shift. Consider the following possibility:

> *Cancer is not a cellular error. 1) It appears for reasons related to chronic stress that forces a person into a survival state, until they can resolve the stress. 2) Cancer does not disappear until that stress (the root cause) is resolved.*

At this point, you may struggle with the idea that cancer is not a 'cellular error'. However, I can assure you that I am not the only one who has worked very closely with cancer patients – getting to know them, their life, their past and their plans for the future – and come to realize that cancer is being triggered by complex factors related to life-challenges. In his book, *Cancer is NOT a Disease*, Andreas Moritz (a prominent naturopath, who has case histories of clients reversing their cancer without using any treatments) states:

> "The possibility that cancer is a survival mechanism has never been considered in the past and is not part of the cancer discussion today. This has had, and still has, fatal consequences."[26]

If what I am saying about cancer is true – that chronic stress pushes our body into survival mode, which triggers cancer growth – your next question might be: "What are the sources of physical, mental, emotional, and spiritual stress that trigger the development of cancer cells, and what can I do to address them?" As you read, you'll learn answers to these questions.

☰ Suggested Article

National post: Is the war on cancer an "utter failure?": A sobering look at how billions in research money is spent. March 15, 2013

https://nationalpost.com/news/war-on-cancer

ROOT CAUSE PRACTITIONER TRAINING

Thank you for the amazing class today, I feel so honored to be able to participate in your course – it's literally what the world needs.

As a western-trained physician, I have observed both professionally and personally, the need for approaching physical illness and disease through a more holistic and empowered lens.

I was telling a close friend today how much I'm enjoying this course, and I don't want it to end! I wish I came across your work a year ago, as I just lost a dear soul to cancer, and he had been searching for 3 years for healing. I met him at a meditation conference as he was researching alternative modalities.

It's really healing just being in the group and having you guide us into our learning. It's clear to me that cancer is not what society has labeled to be a "disease", and what you are offering is a comprehensive and compassionate understanding of what we have called "cancer".

Thank you again – so much appreciation.

Rachel, Medical Doctor

2

YOUR BODY DOESN'T LIE

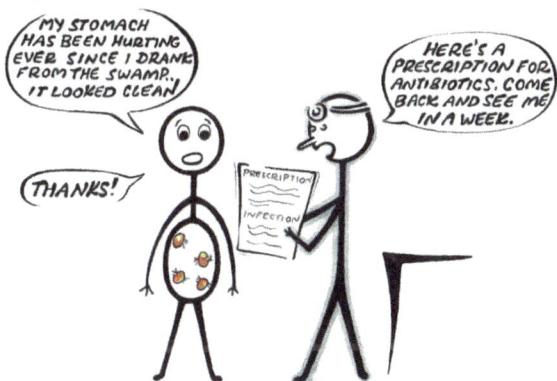

1 WEEK LATER

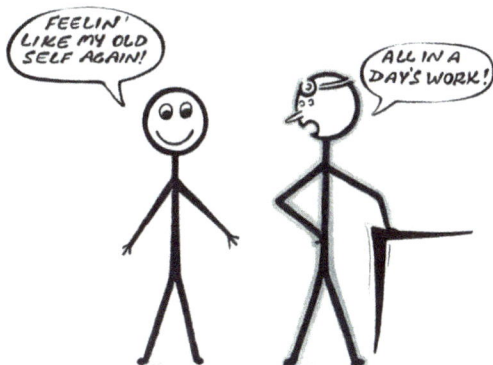

If simply destroying cancer was the answer, you would not be reading this book – cancer would be history.

Historically, some infections, such as gangrene, have been treated by destroying harmful bacteria with antibiotics.

However, applying this "attack and destroy" strategy to cancer has not had the same benefits. For decades, the same mainstream approaches to cancer have been surgery, chemotherapy, and radiation – despite the rising incidence and mortality of cancer. These approaches also have devastating side effects that are so severe that **many patients die not from cancer, but from their treatments.**[27] [28] [29] [30] [31]

The development of chronic diseases like diabetes, heart disease and cancer are directly related to the patient's lifestyle or life circumstances. However, doctors are not extensively trained to investigate life circumstances and stressors, or provide remedial instructions to correct any imbalances or challenges in a patient's life. Doctors have instead become specialists in diagnosing diseases and prescribing drugs matched to the patient's symptoms. The average patient sees their doctor for just fifteen minutes and walks away with a prescription[32] – directly back into the life circumstances that brought them to the doctor in the first place.

The only way to effectively address chronic disease with lasting results is by identifying and resolving complex stress-factors in a person's life. Chronic disease must be healed from within through positive change (and thus cannot be accomplished through some outside force such as a "cure"), and the requirements for self-healing are far more difficult and beyond the basic recommendations for health such as, "exercise and eat healthy". Often, this basic advice may not even be helpful at all – for example, there are endless opinions today about what it means to "eat healthy".

Nonetheless, once our needs are truly met, our body can complete its natural healing process. Some of these needs are: being well-hydrated, sleeping solidly through the night, being well-nourished from consistent organic whole-food meals, freedom, experiencing happiness regularly, and living a purposeful, meaningful life. These examples are so essential for health and healing that if you were to entirely remove any one of them from a person's life, it would threaten their very survival. You will thoroughly learn about all of our human needs, which must be fulfilled to ensure health, healing, and a cancer-free life, in the *What's in a Tear* Series.

> *To heal, we must shift our focus from treating symptoms to the fulfillment of our needs.*

Your body knows how to heal and does so when it is properly supported by your overall lifestyle and life circumstances. For example, if you accidentally cut your finger, your body will heal itself – it will clean and close the wound, rebuilding new tissue, automatically. Now, imagine if you are cut in the same spot chronically – day after day. Your body could not complete its healing, or heal fast enough; pain and other symptoms would rise and the wound would gradually worsen until you would find yourself in a serious crisis (your could lose your finger).

Every day, millions of people are taking drugs in search of relief from some kind of chronic pain or stress – an indication of a repetitive "wounding" of some kind. A human being can be wounded physically and emotionally. For now, let's consider a physical example of a "wound": sleep-deprivation. Ongoing sleep deprivation can lead to any number of symptoms in your body (and mind), such as headaches, low energy, and stressful emotions. A painkiller might relieve the headache, but sleep is what you would need; sleep is how your body and mind repair and regenerate. In the long run, attempting to use a drug as a solution, rather than fulfilling the need (sleep), often leads only to more symptoms and pain.

What if stress (mental, emotional and spiritual) can cause a physical wound in your body? What if chronic, unresolved stress can lead to the development of cancer?

In the book, "The Body Electric", Robert Becker, MD, and Gary Seldon share the following:

> *"Drugs have become the best or only valid treatment for all ailments. Prevention, nutrition, exercise, lifestyle, the patient's physical and mental uniqueness, environmental pollutants [and mental-emotional stress]- all were glossed over [in standard medical education/training]. Even today after so many years and millions of dollars spent for negligible results, it's still assumed that the cure for cancer will be a chemical that kills malignant cells without harming the healthy ones."* [33]

To make real improvements in the incidence and mortality rates of cancer, we need to be willing to look at, and understand, what is going on behind a cancer diagnosis; we need to know what has triggered the development of cancer in each individual situation. If we follow the wise words of Dr. William Osler:

"The good physician treats the disease. The great physician treats the patient who has the disease." [34]

Your body doesn't lie. Pain or any other kind of symptom is your body's way of communicating with us, telling us that something is out of balance, missing, or harmful to us; that something needs to be changed in the way we are eating, drinking, moving, breathing, sleeping or dealing with life-challenges.

A drug that gives relief by blocking the messages of pain, shuts down our body's feedback system. If we want to find the cause of our symptoms, we need to pay close attention to when those symptoms appear and what they are associated with.

Once the root cause of the problem is identified and addressed, the symptoms disappear because the message was heeded and balance restored. This is how our body's feedback system is naturally designed to work – it helps protect us from moving too far out of alignment or into the "wrong direction".

TIP
An efficient and inexpensive way to keep track of your symptoms is to write them in a diary. You may very soon discover patterns like:

- When I eat gluten or refined sugar, my stomach is likely to become bloated.
- When I stay up late I often have a headache, low energy, or a poor mood the next day.
- When I spend too much time with a particular person or neglect my own personal freedom, I feel drained of energy.

If you need help interpreting the messages behind your symptoms, a good health coach can be of great benefit. Ideally, they don't only work on identifying the root cause of your symptoms – they also guide you through a positive-change process, in which you gain more independence, become more in tune with your body, and gain more control over your health and life. If you've found a good coach, you'll know because you will eventually no longer need them.

For advanced education on physical and emotional healing for the prevention of cancer and self-healing, see:

Root Cause Practitioner Training/Course
www.rootcauseinstitute.com

LORNA'S CANCER REVERSAL

My oncologist had given up after years of treatments using chemotherapy, radiation, and surgery. I had Stage 4 cancer that was "terminal" – cancer had spread to my spinal cord. I was told I'd be in a wheelchair within 2 months, and would not survive much longer after that.

Now, eight years later, after seeing Paul at Wheel of Life and applying what I learned, I'm happy to say that I am far from being in a wheelchair. I've gained back 30 pounds and my life has completely transformed. Paul – thank you for helping me gain back control of my life and cancer!

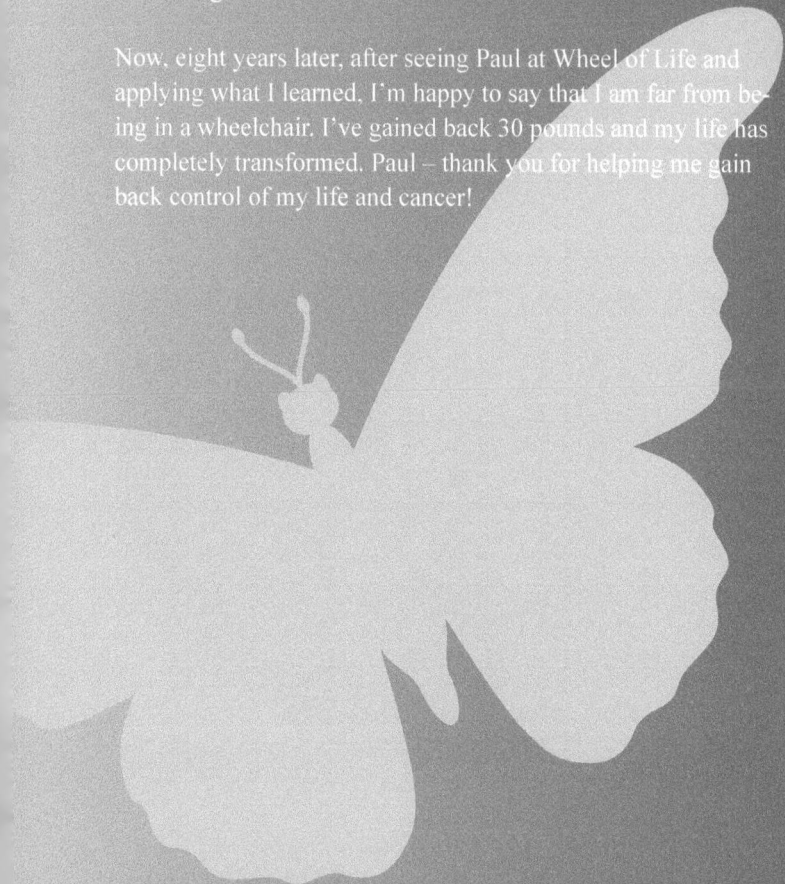

3

ENDING THE WAR ON CANCER

We have technology that allows us to explore the Galaxy in great detail. We have fully functional computers that are so tiny they can barely be seen when placed on the surface of a penny,[35] and we have mapped the human genome. Yet, after trillions of dollars and nearly a century pursuing a method to destroy cancer, we have not accomplished US President Nixon's objective – we have no medical cure.

36

As of 2018, the Canadian Cancer Society celebrated its 80th birthday: 80 years of researching the same approaches to cancer.[37] After all of this time, when subjected to scientific scrutiny, the actual success rates of treatments are appalling: **Chemotherapy for instance, has been documented to have a success rate of just five percent.**[38]

In this picture, notice the date of this LIFE magazine cover, in the bottom right-hand corner (1958!).

LIFE

FRESH HOPE ON CANCER
12 PAGES ON THE NEWEST METHODS
TO SAVE YOU FROM MALIGNANCIES

2,000,000 VOLT
RADIATION FOR
CANCER PATIENT

MAY 5, 1958   25 CENTS

As mentioned, half of Canadians will be diagnosed with cancer in their lifetime, and of those, 50% will die within 5 years, despite treatments. This means 50% will be recorded as "cancer survivors", but cancer statistics are only based on a 5-year survival period.[40] What this means is that if a person is alive 5 years after they were originally diagnosed, **they are recorded as a survivor even if they still have cancer.** Additionally, even if a patient dies of cancer 5-years-and-one-day after their diagnosis, they are still recorded as a cancer survivor.[41] **Hence, the true survival rate of cancer is likely much worse than it appears,** especially since it's so common for a person's cancer to redevelop despite previously being declared cancer-free after treatments.[42]

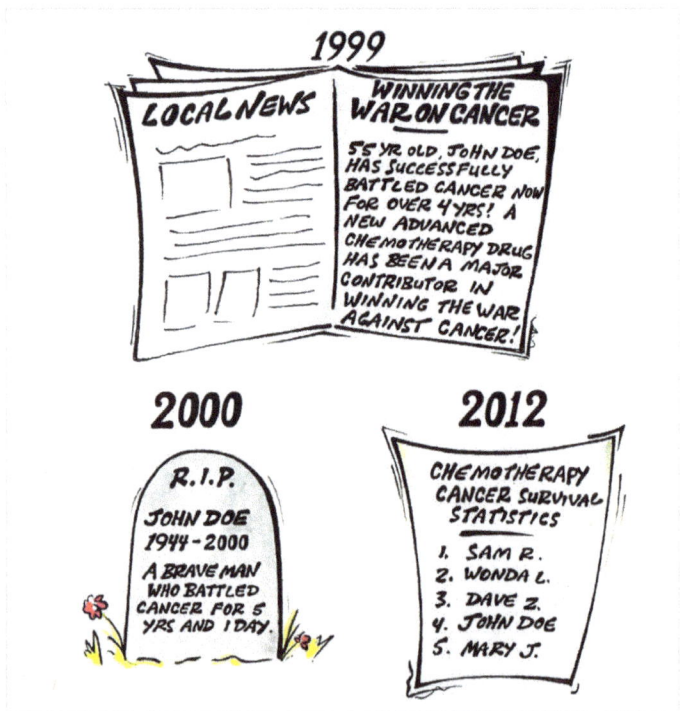

Research on methods for becoming cancer-free outside of chemotherapy, radiation, and surgery are not a priority in the war on cancer.[43] Spontaneous remissions for example (when a person's cancer disappears without any treatments) seems unworthy of significant investigation. Alternative approaches to cancer are defined as "therapy used in place of conventional treatments". Only conventional treatments are considered the "credible", "scientific", and "acceptable" approaches.[44]

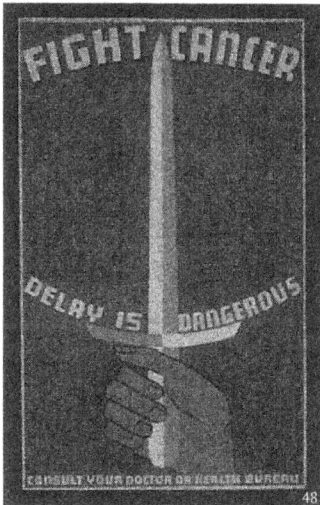

Adopting a new, mainstream approach to overcoming cancer (one that is not focused on destroying cancer cells) is not likely going to be easy: Many corporations have grown into giants, financially fed by the war-mentality towards cancer. The global annual economic cost (and thus profits) of cancer in 2010 is estimated at 1.16 trillion US dollars.[45] Three of the top ten most profitable drugs prescribed by doctors were cancer drugs.[46] There are drugs approved by the FDA that statistically, only increase the survival rate of cancer patients by 12 days, and are sold for $3500 per treatment.[47]

The war approach to cancer began in the early 1900s. In 1936, a radio broadcast was aired to raise money for cancer awareness. The following is an excerpt, with its associated poster.

> "...Our war is to save human life, a war for health and happiness. We are not using bayonets or tanks or machine guns:

Our weapons are leaflets and lectures. We are fighting with facts and our military objectives are the putting to rout of fear and ignorance. This war is against one of the greatest enemies of health. It is against cancer."[49]

How often do you still hear the following statements?
- The war on cancer
- The fight against cancer
- The battle
- Kick cancer's butt
- Fuck cancer
- Someone lost their battle with cancer
- Someone survived their fight with cancer
- There's hope – a cure to win the war is just around the corner

According to Tedx Speaker and Oncologist Dr. Deming and colleagues, whose research was published in the Journal of Psychosocial Oncology: after interviewing 1800 cancer patients their study concluded that 60% of cancer patients found the language of "being a cancer survivor" was not beneficial. In particular, patients reported that the language of "cancer survivor" dismisses four things: the fear of recurrence, the unique experience of each patient, the ongoing struggle after cancer, and it also dismisses the fact that not everyone survives (50%). Additionally, the words "cancer survivor" reminds them of their traumatic time of life, as well as the risk of death from cancer.[50]

Dr. Deming shares open-heartedly in her TEDx Talk about her own mother, who was diagnosed with advanced ovarian cancer, how her family automatically used the language of "battling cancer" with their mother. They said to her, "we're by your side in the fight – soldiers in the battle". But her mother stopped them and she said, "this isn't a fight – I'm healing, and I just want you to love me and pray for me as I heal."

Dr. Deming continues, explaining how "the war on cancer approach" is "great for marketing, but not for healing".[51]

A battle against cancer creates a power struggle and the subtle message is that cancer cannot be overcome by focusing on health principles and positive life changes; only a war – which leads us to look outside ourselves to find something, anything, to destroy cancer for us; a cure, a treatment, a supplement, or maybe a "healer"...

However, if cancer is growing in response to damaging factors present in our lives, then it is the resolution of those factors, that is the real cure.

The growth of cancer is within our control, provided we can look at which parts of our lives and ourselves need to positively transform, in order to address the main sources of unresolved, chronic stress - and then make those changes.

You must become highly motivated to learn how to access your power to heal from within, and you must shed the fears that can prevent you from doing so, by facing them. Then, you can make positive, impactful changes in your life that will deactivate the growth of cancer cells.

There can never be a cure for cancer because cancer cells do not result from an error made within our body. In a way, science has not been failing because winning the war on cancer is impossible; if a focus on health is the only solution for cancer, a "war" simply cannot accomplish that.

The mainstream theory about cancer being a product of a cellular error requires not only one error occurring in a cell, but multiple errors. According to this theory, for a cancer cell to form, a stepwise process must unfold that supposedly involves five consecutive errors, which together lead to the birth of a cancer cell. In *How Cancer Grows*, Lauren Sompayrac states, "Biologists estimate that about five different control systems usually [change] before a cell becomes cancerous."[52] How likely is it that a process involving 5 consecutive steps, which always lead to the same result – a cancer cell – is a series of errors? How could this error-process occur in nearly 50% of humans across the world – any age, race, gender or class, and even in animals? The answer is, it can't!

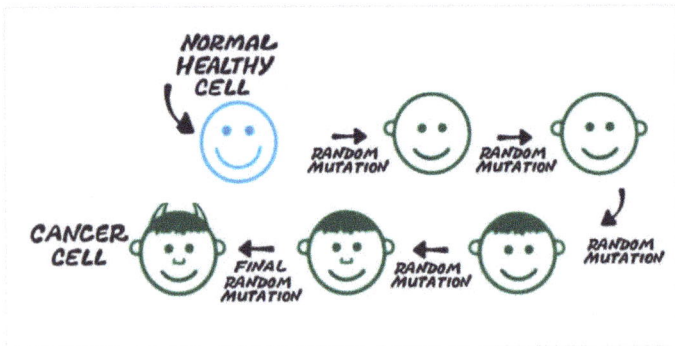

New research indicates that cancer cells resulting from multiple errors are essentially impossible – you read that correctly: impossible. Xialong Meng and colleagues, from the MD Anderson Cancer Center in Houston, report, "If cancer forms from 5 independent point mutations, the theoretical cancer occurrence would be so small that it would be equivalent to the chance of one cancer case in 1.42×10^{23} people. In other words, **no one would develop cancer, in the world**."[53]

> *If the cellular error theory about cancer was correct, mathematically no one would have cancer today.*

Additionally, the cellular-error theory concludes that **our immune system, mistakenly, does not recognize cancer cells as "invaders", hence it never attacks them.**[54] Could it be that our immune system is not attacking cancer cells, because cancer has appeared for a reason?

Is the appearance of cancer an important message that some aspect of our life is not fulfilled to such a degree that **we cannot continue to move forward in wholeness, and we begin "surviving"?** The chronic stress that can build inside our mind and body is so damaging to our physiology that it can destroy parts of our body. **Cancer cells are growing as the result of a survival mechanism which is triggered in response to that stress** – and they can only permanently disappear when that stress is resolved. We must work with cancer, by interpreting the reason for its appearance in any given individual, and respond with appropriate change in ourselves, and our lives.

Research has uncovered the fact that the average person has cancer inside their body for seven years before a formal diagnosis.[55] Despite having cancer, people can live pain and symptom-free for years. Researchers have even concluded that every single person has cancer cells inside their body, every day of their lives.[56] Cancer cells become a problem only if they begin to multiply in numbers so large that they interfere with the function of parts of our body (and this can, and does happen, in the later stages of cancer development). What needs to be answered then is: "Why do some people's cancer cells grow quickly and in large numbers, while others do not?"

Our immune system, which is devoted to the health of our body, does not attack cancer cells.[57] Perhaps it does not (or cannot) for a reason: he root cause of an individual's cancer needs to be identified, understood, and resolved through positive life-changes.

You have likely heard that unlucky genetics are the cause of cancer. Not according to Bruce Lipton, PhD, one of the world's leading researchers in epigenetics. According to Lipton, only 5% or less of all disease is genetic in origin.[58]

Consider research on identical twins – who share the same genes – yet do not have identical cancers.[59] Perhaps what's most revealing is that the risk of cancer in adopted children mirrors that of the families which raised them, but NOT the biological parents.[60] These findings could not be possible if the development of cancer were related to genetics.

In my Root Cause Practice, I have observed that **the real underlying factors correlated with the development of cancer passed on in families, are the factors which perpetuate or elevate chronic stress.** Examples are: coping with stress, how fears are dealth with, connection and communication skills, belief systems, how emotional pain is processed, how to love and care for oneself, how to love others, etc. Unfortunately, most of society does not know how to address or resolve these factors adequately, since our upbringing, school, and society at large does not prepare us for them, or teach us the tools necessary for successfully navigating them. These deeper factors can lead to significant life challenges, such as unresolved stress in relationships or career, which cause significant stress to accumulate in our whole being (body, mind and emotions).

This is why after 15 years of working on the Root Cause of Cancer, I have developed my Real Self Process© taught in my Root Cause Practitioner Training - a life-navigation tool we can use to meet the stressful challenges of life and transcend them (grow through them), rather than get 'stuck' in them.

Cancer appears for a reason, and its "cure" (and prevention) has been here all along. Essentially, it is the resolution of chronic stress.

ROOT CAUSE PRACTITIONER TRAINING

"Hi Paul. I just had to share with you the impact this course is having on me. I literally listen for an hour and sit with myself because, wow, what a journey I've been on.

You have helped me understand my emotions around my cancer diagnosis, what I've been carrying that I couldn't put a finger on. A dark burden, lifted through tears, and time, and realisations.

I have never connected to self in such a beautiful way. I am so in love with my soul right now. With self. With me.

You've given me clarity in so so many ways."

-Shelley

"I am incredibly grateful that I had the opportunity to take your Root Cause Practioner 1 and 2 classes. They changed my life in ways I never thought possible."

-Suzanne

"After taking your class and doing the emotional healing techniques that come with it, my breast cancer just dissolved on it's own and went away."

-Jeanna

"I am extremely grateful that I took part in your course. I appreciated your teaching style, knowledge, wisdom, compassion, material shared, and so much more.
Thank you so much."

-Kathleen

4

OUR BODY'S SURVIVAL RESPONSES

You are dependent upon your body to experience life. Work, play, travel, connecting to those you love, and contributing to humanity in your unique way; everything is dependent on the health of your body. Of course, if you can read this book, it means you have a body – you're using it to accomplish this task. Your body supports, protects, and serves you. Understanding your relationship with your body is instrumental to understand cancer.

At any given second, about six billion biochemical reactions are occurring inside your body.[61] As you read these words, your heart contracts and relaxes, and your blood flows. That blood travels to each of the trillions of cells that make up your body[62] without your conscious involvement. Each cell in your body has an entire set of machinery and instructions it uses to carry out its role (contained in DNA).

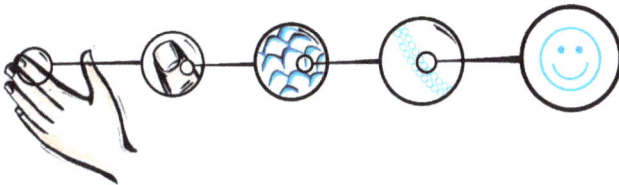

As you navigate life, your body manages the inner workings of your physiology, while you use your mind to make decisions. Every decision you make either supports your body or compromises its function. **Moment to moment, you are either moving towards greater degrees of health and well-being, or towards disease.**

Throughout your life, you are likely to encounter stressful challenges of some kind. If you bump a drink over accidentally and it spills on your cell phone, you'll likely experience mental and emotional stress. That stress can be detrimental to your physiology even though the cause is psychological. Your heart rate and blood pressure would increase, your blood acidity would rise, etc. These blood variables will not return to their normal state until your mind and emotions have stabilized.

Your body's job is to keep you alive and well from the inside out; it is highly adaptable and can deal with a wide range of stress that you may encounter. It clears out toxins you are exposed to, and delivers nutrients (that you choose to ingest!) to your cells after eating a meal. When your body's cells are in a good state, free of toxins and saturated with nutrients, these cells are in a state of 'homeostasis'.[63]

Homeostasis is dependent on the fulfillment of both your physical and psychological needs. If your needs are not met, your body is put under stress of some form, which forces it to attempt to restore balance. If even one cell somewhere in your body begins to lose homeostasis, your body must begin rectifying the situation immediately. And it does – or at least it tries.

Reaching a state of homeostasis results in feeling calm, energized, centered, and happy – it is the state in which you are healing (or healed). For this reason, it is impossible to heal

your body if you are living in a reality that is continually causing you stress, or blocking your ability to fulfill your needs. Your
"outer world" is a direct reflection of your "inner world". If a
large number of cells in your body are overly stressed, entire
parts of your body can fail, and even die. For example, in the
case of a heart attack, cells of the heart have malfunctioned
due to some form of stress that has surpassed the body's ability to recover from.

> *If cancer cells have developed in your body, it means you
> have lost homeostasis as a result of chronic stress in your
> life.*

Each of the cells of our body is nourished by our blood. Thus,
homeostasis is dependent on our bloodstream, moment to
moment – it is one of the most critical aspects of health. To
remain healthy, one of the goals of the body is to keep blood
flowing, delivering life-supporting nutrients to all our cells. Simultaneously, our blood carries away various forms of toxins,
to our detoxification and elimination organs. All of our cells
– bones, muscle, skin, organs, and brain – critically depend on
bloodflow for their ongoing health.

Our blood must have appropriate levels of oxygen, nutrients,
salinity, acidity, temperature, pressure, glucose (sugar), and
more. If any variable becomes imbalanced, homeostasis is lost,
and if this occurs too often, it becomes a threat to our body's
survival.

**Our body responds to the enormous variety of potential stress-
ors by activating one or more of its many automatic survival responses.** Whenever the well-being of our body's cells is threatened, our body "knows" instantly and responds. For example, if

cade of physiological changes: breathing rate increases, heart rate increases, and many blood variables change. Your knee becomes inflamed and swollen – and it is your body that causes the increase in blood flow to that damaged area. This is called inflammation. **Inflammation is our body's choice – its main response to some form of stress (it is not an error).**

The Inflammatory Response is one of the survival-responses of our body, for tending to its damaged or stressed parts. Increased blood flow helps more oxygen and nutrients reach damaged cells; swelling and pain help reduce movement to bring cautious attention to the wounded area. The immune system is also involved, sending specialized cells to the inflamed location to help clean the area and repair or build new cells. Once the knee has been repaired and brought back to homeostasis, the body will deactivate both the inflammatory and immune survival-responses – but not until then.

The most well-known survival response that our body uses is called the "Fight-or-Flight Response", also known as the "Stress-Response", [64] which is covered in greater detail in Chapter 6.

To begin to understand cancer we need to recognize that **every survival-response has associated drawbacks.** For example, the inflammatory response causes pain, and the pain can become so great that it feels unbearable; we can even lose consciousness, which is also a threat to our survival.

If a survival-response occurs temporarily, it means we have only experienced acute stress. Conversely, if any survival-response in our body is activated continuously, it means our body is in an ongoing threatened state. **Sooner or later, a chronic stress state will lead to disease.**

The reason chronic stress leads to disease is because of two main reasons: One is that u**our body can only survive for so long without your needs met.** For example, you cannot survive long without consuming clean water, because water is a **need**.

The other reason is due to **the damaging effects of the various survival-responses, which our body must use to extend life.** Survival-responses come at a cost to the body because they use up its vital energy and resources.

> *Our body does everything it can to function optimally at all times. Whenever any cell is in trouble, our body becomes stressed and responds by activating one or more survival responses.*

More examples of survival responses in your body:

Low Temperature
Our internal blood temperature must remain around 98.6 degrees F.[65] If our bloodstream becomes too hot or cold, it will activate a survival-response. For example, when threatened by cold, our body responds by developing goosebumps on the skin, and by redirecting blood flow. Goosebumps cause a thin airspace to form between bumps. The airspace creates a layer of insulation between the outside cold air and your skin, which slows heat loss from the body. Additionally, blood vessels near our extremities constrict, and blood vessels near the center of our body dilate. This forces warm blood to circulate more to the core parts of our body, prioritizing the survival of organs. This redirection grants us extra time to solve the temperature-related threat.

As mentioned earlier, each survival-response has drawbacks. In this example, while blood becomes more concentrated around vital organs, our skin and extremities become more vulnerable to the cold, making them more susceptible to frostbite. What can our body do? It has no choice but continue to divert blood away from our fingers and extremities even though they also need warm blood to survive.

High Temperature

If our body temperature becomes too high, it is also a threat to our survival. To survive extreme heat, our body activates the survival-response of sweating. The evaporation of water from the surface of our skin causes a cooling effect. However, as our body is forced to release water, the risk of dehydration rises. Sweating allows us to survive extreme heat longer than otherwise, but until we solve the temperature crisis, our body will be forced to continuously dehydrate itself.

Starvation

We must eat food to acquire a wide assortment of nutrients to support the health of each of our cells. When our nutrient or energy stores get low, our body communicates with us through the sensation of hunger: it "tells us" to eat. We chew and swallow food which enters our stomach and is liquefied by strong acids. The food then enters our intestines, where its nutrients are absorbed into our bloodstream.

TIP 1

If you experience the sensation of hunger and then proceed to eat food that lacks nutrition, you can easily overeat and end up feeling full, yet unsatisfied. This is common with commercial foods because they are grown on nutrient-depleted soil due to poor farming practices. Additionally, many of the so-called "foods" available for consumption today are not food – rather, they are some kind of food-like product laced with addictive or artificially attractive substances, containing little to no real food at all.

TIP 2

If you have cancer, eat only when you are hungry. Listen to and trust the body. Sometimes your body may need to fast – it will tell you by not sending you hunger messages. Other times, your body may be ready for food – again, it will tell you when, and how much. Trust your body. If you are without an appetite chronically, then you may need to look into other possible causes such as depression.

Also, pay close attention to the side effects of prescription drugs or treatments, which can cause loss of appetite, because the body must divert its resources to detoxification rather than digestion of food.

On average, a person can live for up to 65 days without eating food before they die of starvation.[66] The starvation survival-response is a process whereby the body begins to digest itself. It consumes parts that are less of a priority, such as fat and muscle, compared to vital organs. It will even digest bones to add minerals to the bloodstream. This process can obviously become problematic. Fat is important for many reasons, such as insulation to maintain body temperature, as well as for storing fat-soluble vitamins. Muscle powers our ability to move, and bones provide stability. However, our body knows that our organs are still more important, and if our organs are not prioritized, we'll die. Thus, our body is forced to consume (metabolize) parts of itself to increase the chance of survival. **Activating the starvation survival-response will hopefully give us enough time to find food.**

Diarrhea

It is well known that when our body develops an infection, especially in the digestive tract, this can lead to diarrhea. Diarrhea is our body's attempt to flush out the problem using water. However, the loss of water simultaneously causes dehydration. Once again, until the root cause is addressed (such as a parasite infection), our body must continue utilizing diarrhea as a survival-response.

Extreme Infection

In circumstances of extreme infection, our immune system responds by not only destroying harmful bacteria, but also surrounding healthy cells.[67] Paul Chek, author of *How to Eat, Move, and Be Healthy*, describes this drastic immune response using the analogy of "throwing a grenade" into the area of infection. To increase the speed at which the infection can be eradicated, the immune system must make a compromise, which is the sacrifice of healthy cells along with the harmful bacteria. If the infection is not resolved soon enough, the body can destroy localized areas, as it attempts to eliminate the infection.

Fatigue

When our energy levels get too low, our body forces us to fall asleep, which conserves vital energy for organs. Even when we are in life-threatening situations, such as being out in the wilderness at night with potential threats around, we will still succumb to sleep if we run out of energy. This survival-response automatically shuts down our entire system to keep us alive!

Cancer

Cancer may be the result of a complex survival-response, serving a purpose along with its own set of side effects – side effects which can lead to death, if the underlying issue is not addressed. Chronic stress can lead to significant cell damage in our body from excess blood glucose, and unhealthy diet and lifestyle factors can also contribute to, or escalate the damage. **Cancer cells absorb substantial amounts of blood glucose,**[68] which would otherwise damage or destroy parts of your body. Could cancer be protecting a localized part of our body from excess glucose damage?

> *Cancer may be the result of a survival response that our body uses to give us more time to resolve the main source(s) of stress in our life, by reducing damage to particular areas of our body in the meantime.*

DONNA'S CANCER REVERSAL

Finding the root cause of my cancer was very important to me. I am a holistic nutritionist and I knew intuitively that my cancer came from much more than my diet and environment.

After speaking with Paul, I decided to work one-on-one with him. I wanted to understand what emotions and behaviours were causing me to create dis-ease in my body. I learned how important it was to have a dialogue with myself, to spend the time alone and discover more about myself.

Paul was very easy to work with and he helped me find those ah-ha moments. Paul guided me through the steps of self healing and emotional processing. I continually review the steps and practice of self dialogue to make sure I am not repeating the past behaviours.

It has been almost a year since my diagnosis and subsequent surgery. I have embarked on a natural course of healing and I feel a big part of my cancer staying in remission is from the work I did with Paul. I will continue to do the work to assist my body in maintaining optimal health and will always live my life with gratitude in my heart.

5

MANAGING BLOOD GLUCOSE

One of the most important blood variables your body must manage is glucose. Glucose is the scientific term for a type of sugar in the bloodstream. It's normal and necessary to have glucose in the bloodstream, but if glucose levels become too high or low, it threatens the survival of our body. Any diabetic will tell you that if your body loses the ability to effectively manage glucose concentrations, it is life-threatening.

Glucose is an important component of our bloodstream – it is one of the main fuels for our cells. This is why if it gets too low, our cells begin to starve, malfunction, and die. **If blood glucose gets too high, the excess concentration in our bloodstream draws water out of the cells of our body, which dehydrates and destroys them.**[69] Surges in glucose can cause damage to all systems of our body, including the neurological, cardiovascular, and reproductive systems, the retina of the eyes, the kidneys, and more.[70] If excess blood glucose occurs chronically, disease will develop in our body.

William Dufty, the author of "Sugar Blues", explains:

> *"Excess sugar [in your diet] eventually affects every organ in the body... A daily intake of refined sugar soon makes the liver expand like a balloon, and tissues degenerate and turn to fat. The whole body is then affected by their reduced ability, and abnormal blood pressure is created... The quality of*

red corpuscles starts to change... tolerance and immunizing power becomes more limited, and teeth and bone deteriorate. [Chronic excess blood sugar] leads to symptoms of crippling, and worldwide diseases such as diabetes, cancer, and heart illnesses." [71]

Regulating blood glucose is so critical that our body has an entire organ, the pancreas, primarily devoted to keeping glucose levels balanced. If levels are chronically out of balance, parts of the body begin to die – it is a very serious situation. Diabetics are known to lose their toes, feet, and even their legs, due to chronic low blood glucose. More than 11 million Canadians have diabetes or pre-diabetes (That is almost a third of the entire population of Canada).[72]

A healthy pancreas releases the hormone "glucagon" when glucose levels drop; this triggers the release of stored glucose from liver cells and other cells throughout the body, raising blood glucose back to normal.

If glucose surges beyond safe levels, the pancreas releases the hormone "insulin" which triggers the opposite effect, causing our cells to absorb glucose from the bloodstream, thereby lowering it.

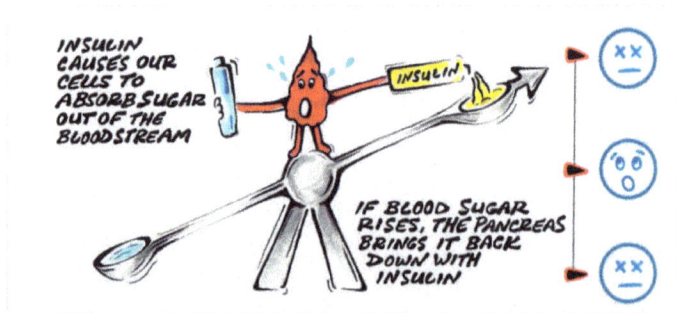

INSULIN CAUSES OUR CELLS TO ABSORB SUGAR OUT OF THE BLOODSTREAM

INSULIN

IF BLOOD SUGAR RISES, THE PANCREAS BRINGS IT BACK DOWN WITH INSULIN

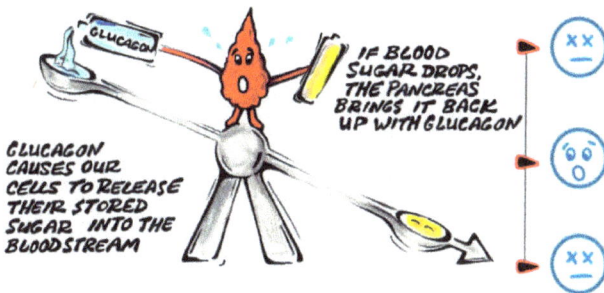

NOTE: Cancer cells have a special ability to absorb glucose from the bloodstream (see chapter 7).

Our pancreas, using glucagon and insulin as explained, monitors and manages blood glucose concentration.

When chronic or extreme glucose fluctuations occur, the pancreas, whether healthy or not, cannot likely restore blood glucose balance fast enough to avoid some degree of cellular damage or death.

Two main factors can cause damaging high elevations of glucose: physical factors like eating a diet high in refined sugar, and the psychological factors of stress, related to life-challenges.[73]

TIP

To lose weight, some conventional ideas suggest cutting out fat, counting calories, and doing regular cardiovascular exercise. If it were that simple, obesity statistics wouldn't be so high. Firstly, refined sugar is one of the main culprits of excess weight gain because of it's addictive qualities. Fat consumption is not the problem – we need healthy fats in our diet for many reasons, but we do not need refined sugar at all.

Radical behaviour of children is often diagnosed as ADHD (Attention Deficit Hyperactivity Disorder). One of the main causes or contributing factors of ADHD is that many children are fed processed foods that cause surges in glucose due to high concentrations of refined sugar. As a result, children often become hyperactive, which is an effective way to burn up excess

glucose from their bloodstream. Psychologically, children often become hyperactive because they need attention. Unfortunately, the root of the problem is often misunderstood and not addressed. Rather than focusing on improving a child's diet and connecting with their soul to see what kinds of freedom they need (part of a healthy childhood), or how much attention they need from parents and adults (the evidence to a child that they matter). Children need to connect with nature - not screens, and this has also led to an increase in ADHD. Instead, many children are prescribed pharmaceutical drugs.

From birth, children are extremely vulnerable to our society's current crisis of health. Unfortunately, many parents are un-aware of the extent to which many common "foods" damage their children. The average person tends to first trust all that is provided to the public by large "food" manufacturing corpo-rations. However, there are plenty of companies whose main goal is making money – not the provision of life-supporting, nutrition for children, and they don't care what the cost is to the consumer for eating their attractive products.

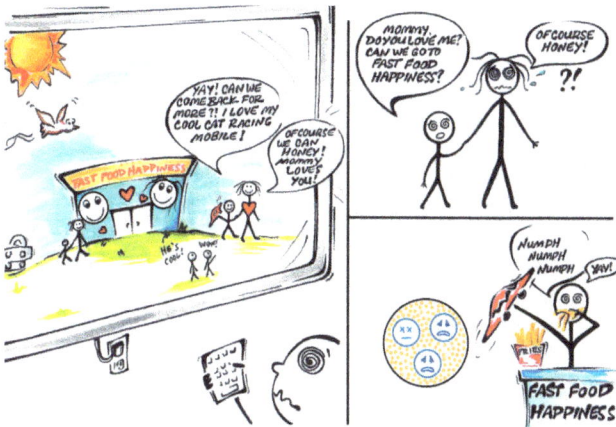

The business of selling sugar and chemical-based "foods" to the public (especially children) is incredibly lucrative. **Heavy marketing exists to get you to consume what is not even good for you, or will cause disease in your body.** Part of healing means learning about this and paying attention to what kind of information you allow yourself to be exposed to because it is designed to influence your values and the choices you make. To heal or prevent cancer, you must establish your own values that truly nourish you, and set clear boundaries to ensure you live by them.

Considering the fact that cancer cells absorb excess glucose from the bloodstream, once an individual accomplishes adopting a lifestyle that results in consistent blood glucose balance, they'll have mastered one of the most critical factors for the prevention (and reversal) of cancer, and simultaneously, fulfilled factors that sustain and create overall health.

TIP
It is essential to understand that any advertisements, marketing, or "scientific" studies that steer you away from eating whole organic food, most likely don't have your best interests in mind.

Many "foods" today, cause excessive blood glucose surges. Prior to 1800, the only foods commonly available were actual foods such as apples, carrots, broccoli, potatoes, lettuce, cucumbers and so on. Factory farming did not exist: animals were generally healthy and happy throughout their life before their death (raised outside, eating a diet that was natural for them). These types of whole foods generally do not cause the levels of blood sugar spikes that we see prevalent in the mainstream Western diet today, and this is why it is important to be particularly careful about the types of food you ingest.

In the next chapter, we'll look at the fight-or-flight system, and how **blood sugar can rise from our minds alone.**

ROOT CAUSE COACHING

Paul, I can't quite put into words what our call meant to me today. I feel as though you changed my life just by giving me knowledge and power over my mind, thoughts and emotions. Thank you so much. I look forward to more sessions with you.
-Kellie

I am loving my healing journey and I've fallen back in love with life again, and even when I"m not feeling right I turn to your videos, meditations and music, and I know I'm healing.
-Karen

I can't find the words right now to express how grateful I am for our session yesterday and what has transpired since then... God bless you for the beautiful human being that you are and the amazing work you're doing!
Thank you.
-Silvia

Thank you for our session two weeks ago. I really appreciated your additional insight on my situation.

Now I have big waves of "positive" emotions like joy and gratitude that make me cry! I really didn't know I was suppressing SO MUCH FEELING!!

With gratitude,
Claire

6

FIGHT OR FLIGHT

We have discussed how threats to homeostasis trigger different survival responses in our body, and the damaging effect elevated blood glucose has on cells in our body. Now, let's look a little closer at the Fight-or-Flight System, which is our body's main psychological survival response; also called the Stress Response.

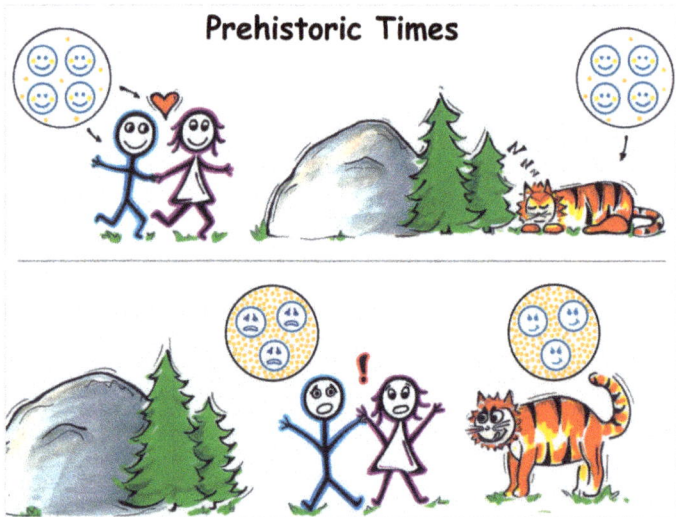

Prehistoric Times

The Stress Response increases our chances of surviving threatening situations that you encounter with our mind, by quickly mobilizing large amounts of stored glucose into our blood-

stream, from our liver and other cells of our body. The surge of glucose fuels our brain and musculoskeletal system, temporarily heightening our alertness and ability to fight or escape threats when needed. Hence, our body has sufficient time to recover.

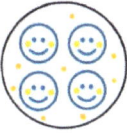

SUGAR MOLECULE

HOMEOSTASIS

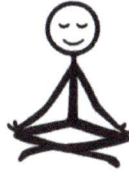

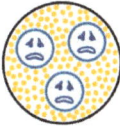

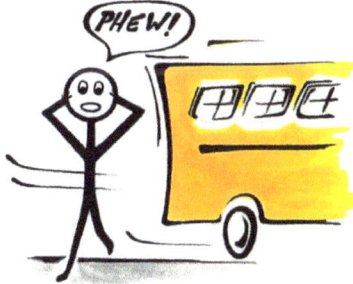

PHEW!

30 MINUTES LATER

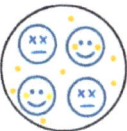

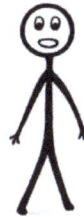

The Stress Response is part of our DNA – we cannot separate ourselves from it. For example, if you accidentally step in front of a bus and come within inches of being hit, you'll automatically experience the side effects of an immense Stress Response: Your heart rate will increase dramatically, and your legs will be trembling because stress hormones and glucose flooded your bloodstream. The good thing is, you safely avoided the bus. The bad thing is, the Stress Response comes with a cost: that surge of glucose may have damaged or even destroyed some of the cells in your body. However, you will recover from the stressful event because you probably don't step in front of buses on a regular basis (if you do, you need to start paying attention!).

The Stress Response is governed by our Nervous System, which has two opposing branches: the sympathetic and parasympathetic. The sympathetic branch is what floods our bloodstream with glucose, waking us up and energizing our body – temporarily heightening our alertness and physical capabilities. The parasympathetic branch does the opposite: it calms us down, lowers blood glucose to normal levels, and puts our body into a regenerative healing state to restore homeostasis. The two branches work in opposition – the more one branch is active, the less the other and vice versa. In other words, **our body cannot be in a state of stress and breakdown, and at the same time be in a state of peace and regeneration.**

During the 1920s, pioneering scientist Hans Selye, who is considered the "Father of the Stress Response", discovered that an organism's ability to resist stressors is always limited; health breaks down as stress persists.[74] When stress persists, it causes chronic activation of the Stress Response, which has serious consequences: It prevents the parasympathetic system from doing its regenerative healing work, and simultaneously keeps the sympathetic branch active along with its detrimental side effects. Thus, chronic stress is a serious threat to our well-being.

One way to get a sense for how much chronic stress is experienced today by most people, is by looking at adrenal gland health. The more stress a person has been under, without sufficient time to regenerate, the weaker their adrenal glands will be. According to James Wilson in his book *Adrenal Fatigue: The 21st Century Stress Syndrome*, during stress, a part of the brain (the hypothalamus) releases corticotropic-releasing hormone (CRH). CRH causes the pituitary gland to release Adrenocorticotropic Hormone (ACTH), which travels through the bloodstream and attaches to the adrenal glands – two small "stress-organs" located on top of the kidneys. ACTH triggers the adrenal glands to release Cortisol and Epinephrine into the bloodstream; these two stress-hormones stimulate blood glucose to surge.[75] The significant degree of chronic stress today has resulted in 80% of [United States] adults suffering from adrenal fatigue.[76]

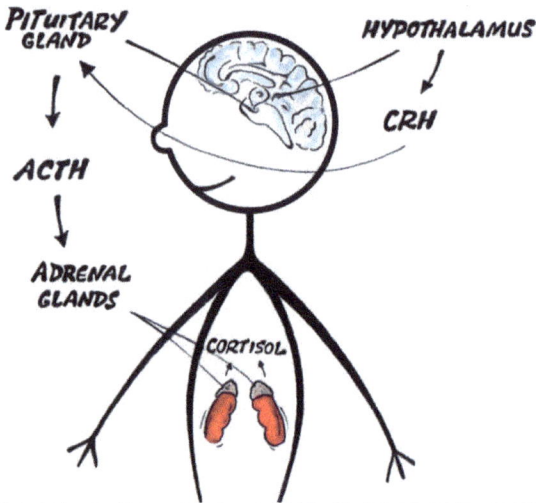

When the Stress Response is triggered, our blood vessels become flooded with glucose. First, glucose is transported to muscles to energize them for movement to respond to the perceived threat. Afterwards, blood is redistributed evenly throughout our body (An exception to this is in the case of inflamed areas in the body, which will be discussed in the next chapter). Gradually, our body lowers excess blood glucose after stress by reabsorbing it.

Today, the Fight-or-Flight Stress Response is often triggered without any real physical threat – we are rarely chased by tigers. Thus, **when the Stress Response is activated and no significant physical movement results (such as running away or fighting), the surge in blood glucose is not quickly burned up as fuel.** This likely intensifies the damage done by excess blood glucose. Here is an example: if a stressed secretary's body is flooded with glucose, it will cause damage to her physiology; but additional damage occurs because her fingers typing on a keyboard can't possibly burn up the surge of glucose.

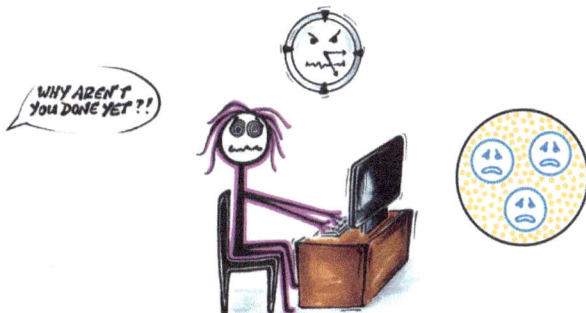

In addition to the glucose damage caused by the initial Stress-Response, damage continues to occur after the event is over: Research shows that after a stress-episode, **stress hormones continue to circulate in the bloodstream for several hours.**[77]

These are some of the ways in which the side effects of the Stress Response lead to significant glucose damage in your body.

In the early 1900s, famous researcher Walter Cannon and colleagues at Harvard University, conducted a major study on the Stress Response, which uncovered an important interplay between emotions, stress hormones and blood glucose.[78] Cannon found that when a cat was strapped into a holder and exposed to a barking dog, significant quantities of epinephrine [a stress hormone] suddenly appeared in the cat's bloodstream. He also found large quantities of glucose appeared in the cat's urine.

Taking his research further, Cannon took urine samples from Harvard students amid stressful exams, and with striking frequency students had excess glucose in their urine.

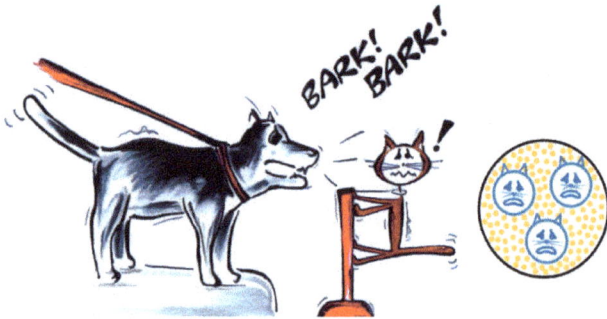

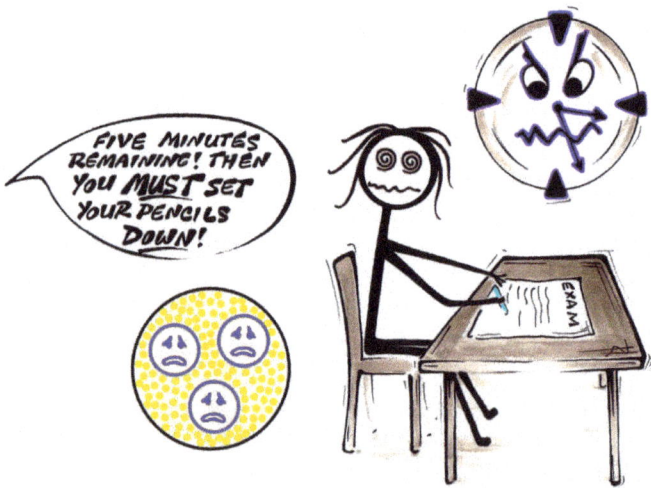

Cannon went to the Harvard football field and collected urine from players during the most exciting game of the season: even players sitting on the bench had elevated glucose concentrations, compared to the players that were on the field.[80]

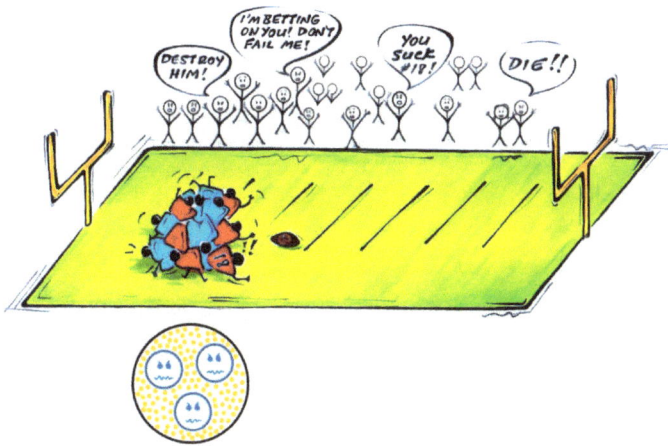

A concerning study carried out by Dr. Lennart Levi of the Caroline Institute in Stockholm, showed that there was more than enough stress in some jobs to continually cause sharp rises in blood sugar. He devised an experiment in which he duplicated the irritation and boredom inherently found in many factory jobs, giving volunteers the tedious task of sorting 2000 steel balls that were similar in size. The boredom and stress of the job was worsened by harassment from noise, bright light, criticisms, and a tight deadline. As you can guess, epinephrine (and blood sugar) levels rose sharply.[81]

Our body's instinctive focus on survival ensures we are always responding to threats. **The Stress Response will continue to activate no matter how much damage accumulates in our body as a result.** If it did not, our body would risk not surviving threats when they occur. Imagine stepping in front of a bus, and your Stress Response did not activate to give you the boost of energy and alertness you needed to jump out of the way? The problem is, our Survival Response should only be occurring occasionally – not chronically. Ongoing unresolved

6AM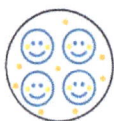

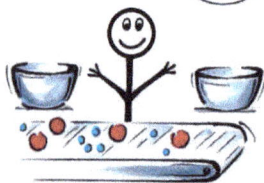

7AM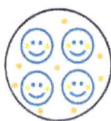

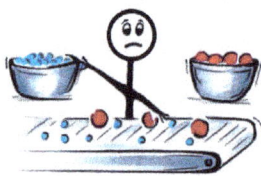

8AM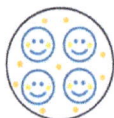

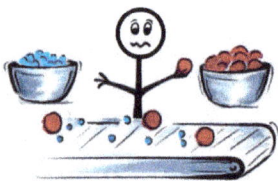

9AM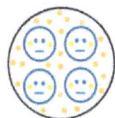

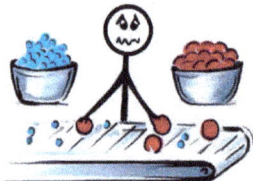

10AM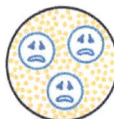

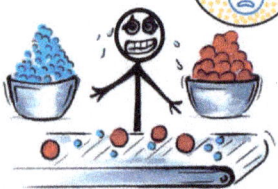

10:01AM - BREAK TIME

Poof!

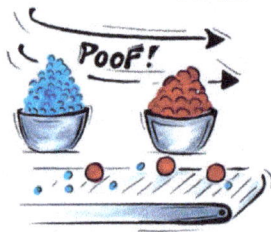

74

stress in a relationship or in some other form of life-challenge, will continue to take a toll on our body.

In *Why Zebras Don't Get Ulcers,* Robert M Sapolsky, a prominent researcher of the Stress Response states:

> *"...Sitting frustrated in traffic jams, worrying about expenses, mulling over tense interactions with colleagues. If you repeatedly turn on the stress-response, or if you cannot turn off the stress-response at the end of an event, it can eventually become damaging. A large percentage of what we think of when we talk about stress-related diseases are the result of excessive stress-responses."[82]*

Sapolsky's book explains that, unlike people, zebras only experience acute, short-term stress, such as being chased by a lion. Hence, they do not suffer the kinds of health challenges common for the average human being today. Zebras are free of the stress that comes with unresolved relationship challenges, worries about money or survival, judgment of self or others, or the pain of feeling like one does not matter. The question is: **if zebras began developing cancer, would we start searching for a cure for them? Or would we investigate what changes have been occurring in the life of the average zebra? (Likewise, for any other animal that develops cancer).**

TIP

To be clear, stress is not a bad thing – only chronic, unresolved stress. Healthy amounts of stress is a normal part of life. For example, physically, your body will become weak without adequate exercise (a form of stress) because muscles deteriorate when unused. If your muscles deteriorate, it places extra responsibility on your heart to pump blood, because the heart normally works synchronistically with them.[83]

In "Vibrational Medicine", Richard Gerber, MD, states the following:

> *"If there were no stress, there would be no growth. Even bone needs some type of stress to maintain its form and strength. If an individual never got out of bed, their bones would begin to re-absorb and weaken so that even the simplest movements would become painful. There is a certain functional amount of stress."* [84]

The ability to navigate through psychological stress is a strength that is important to develop to remain healthy. For example, death is part of life, but facing experiences of death – such as losing a pet, child, parent or partner – can be one of the most psychologically stressful experiences we can ever have; and it can take a toll on our body. **Thus, it is important to develop strength by growing through these experiences, thereby developing what I call spiritual strength.** To be clear, it would be unhealthy to experience losses of this nature, and not feel emotional pain. What's essential, is to learn and grow, and let go, so you don't carry stress for longer than "necessary".

Our mind, if we let it run wild, can destroy our body; just thinking about something stressful can active the Stress Response. [85] Try remembering a stressful experience you've had and notice how your body feels – your blood glucose may rise in this very moment. Imagine what can happen to a person's health due to cellular glucose damage, if they spend months drowning in unresolved psychological stress?

Many different psychological experiences can be stressful and hence damaging to your body: Worry, judgment towards yourself or others, resentment, regret, grief, hatred, anger, rage, anxiety, control, blame, dishonesty, apathy, etc – all have physiological repercussions on your body. Perhaps the most damaging psychological experience is being stuck, chronically, in a

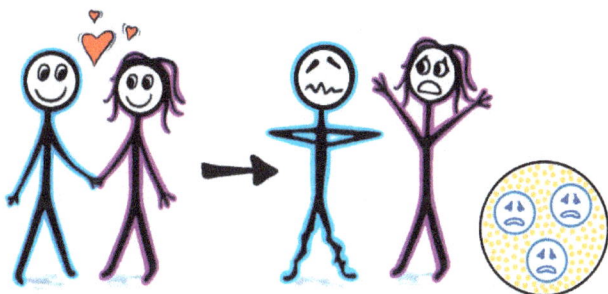

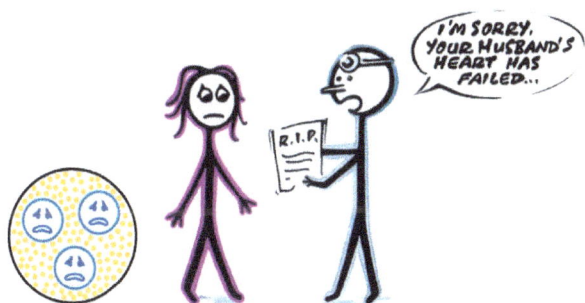

Years Later...

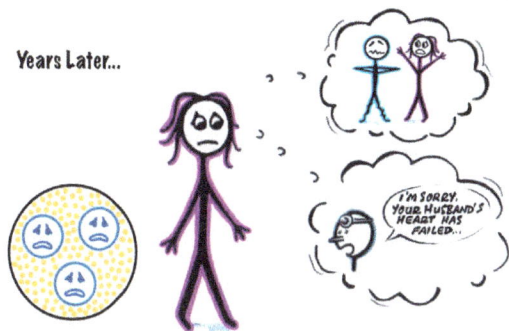

state of fear. **This is why growing through challenges and becoming stronger, spiritually, is essential to create and maintain health, and thrive.** Spiritual growth in this regard, means transforming these painful negative emotions into understanding, empathy, love, acceptance, and ultimately life changes which prevent more negative experiences (more on this in book 2).

Research shows that cancer patients have twice the mental-emotional stress compared to the general population.[86] Therefore, understanding and resolving these kinds of stressors is crucial to prevent or reverse cancer.

(▶) **Suggested Video**
Bozeman science, Fight or Flight Response
www.youtube.com/watch?v=m2GywoS77qc

KRISTEN'S CANCER REVERSAL

I was diagnosed with stage 3 cancer in August, 2017, and my on-cologist gave me two choices: one was surgery to have my spleen taken out and other was a drug called Retuxin. My spleen was so enlarged that it could easily rupture, and both treatments came with a high chance I could die within 24 hours.

I was so scared… and I decided I would not do either treatment. Thankfully, I had the opportunity to meet Paul, and in my second session, we had a very huge breatkthrough. After a few days I could feel a difference in my spleen, and it was obvious to me that it was shrinking. Two weeks later my stomach was so much flatter that I could once again bring my knee to my chest, and put my socks on. Whereas before, I couldn't because it was like I was pregnant, and my belly got in the way.

Paul, thank you, I would not be healed today without you.

7

THE SPECIAL ABILITY OF CANCER CELLS

Over 3.5 trillion dollars are spent on healthcare each year in the United States alone[87] – more than any other country in the world. Yet, the United States has one of the highest rates of cancer and other chronic diseases. On the list of the World's Healthiest Nations, the United States ranks way down at 64th.[88]

Worldwide, every day over 26,000 people die in the War on Cancer.[89] Most choose chemotherapy, radiation, or surgery as their weapons. The others look for natural weapons. **Cancer wins the war 26,000 times a day.**

Recall what Hippocrates, the father of medicine, said about cancer in 400BCE.[90] He believed that too much or too little of any of the "humours" in the body cause disease – specifically, that an excess of black bile caused cancer. Hippocrates' theory was much closer to the truth than today's mainstream theory about cancer – he realized that an imbalance in a person's body can trigger cancer growth.

Today's dominant theory says Hippocrates was wrong, instead asserting that our body has been making cellular errors for more than 2000 years. Our body can't figure out how to stop making the same erroneous cell – a cancer cell – and all the money and scientists in the world cannot find a cure.

> *Today's most common theory about cancer is preventing the majority of humanity from focusing on and resolving the cause of cancer.*

It's difficult not to focus on killing cancer cells when the belief about cancer being a cellular error and a war being needed to solve the problem, are perpetuated decade after decade. All the while, solutions for healing oneself are largely unknown or not taken seriously. This can leave people feeling desperate for outside help (a physical solution) when the real healing is done inside (making changes in one's life).

In the 1970s, during the initial stages of the intensive "War on Cancer", Ronald Herberman, Senior Immunology Branch Investigator of the National Cancer Institute, issued a statement outlining what he believed to be a much-needed change in the approach to studying, understanding, and treating cancer:

> *"We need to understand what fuels cancer and what would lead to its natural destruction within the body. We basically need an entirely new paradigm – not based on cutting, burning and poisoning."[91]*

This is a statement made over 50 years ago, yet, the common approach to cancer today is still focused on cutting, burning, and poisoning! The most deadly medical "weapons" designed by human beings have made the human body a battleground: for instance, chemotherapy is derived from mustard gas which was used as a weapon in World War II,[92] and it is now believed that both chemotherapy and radiation can cause cancer.[93]

In 2008, my stepfather died of lung cancer (this is what set me on my journey of discovering the Root Cause of Cancer). Back then, I had no idea what caused cancer, nor did any of my family, and no one knew how to heal. Nothing was working to heal my stepfather, and his oncologist insisted he started treatments. Just before my stepfather received his first treatment, he said "I'm not sure how I feel about this...", and his oncologist said, "Don't worry, your cells will love you for it". A few weeks later, my stepfather died, and my entire family is absolutely certain that the treatments caused him to die sooner than he would have without them. It was about 2 years later that I realized that unresolved emotional pain was what my stepfather needed help to resolve, in order to heal.

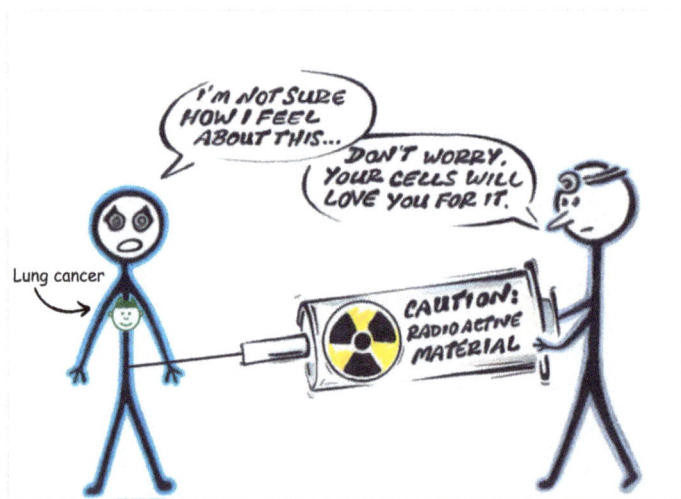

After "successful" treatments, in which cancer patients often suffer from severe poisoning or even lose body parts, they then commonly experience life-long side effects. For example, cancer survivors can suffer from nerve damage called "chemo-associated peripheral neuropathy", that results in pain, tingling, burning, weakness or numbness in their fingers and toes, which can expand into the arms and legs.[94]

"Chemo brain" is a term used for the brain damage that can result from chemotherapy – patients often suffer cognitive problems, including mental fogginess and trouble with concentration, memory and multitasking. Symptoms often last for years, and sometimes a lifetime.[95]

"Late effects" is a term used for the commonly experienced side effects of cancer treatments which can be lifelong. The mayo clinic lists the following side effects of medical treatments for cancer.[96]

Chemotherapy
- Dental problems
- Early menopause
- Hearing loss
- Heart problems
- Increased risk of other cancers
- Infertility
- Loss of taste
- Lung disease
- Nerve damage
- Osteoporosis
- Reduced lung capacity

Radiation
- Cavities and tooth decay
- Early menopause
- Heart and vascular problems
- Hypothyroidism
- Increased risk of other cancers
- Increased risk of stroke

- Infertility
- Intestinal problems
- Lung disease
- Lymphedema
- Memory problems
- Osteoporosis

These outcomes could be avoided if the root cause of cancer in an individual's life were understood and resolved, so that cancer cells could disappear naturally.

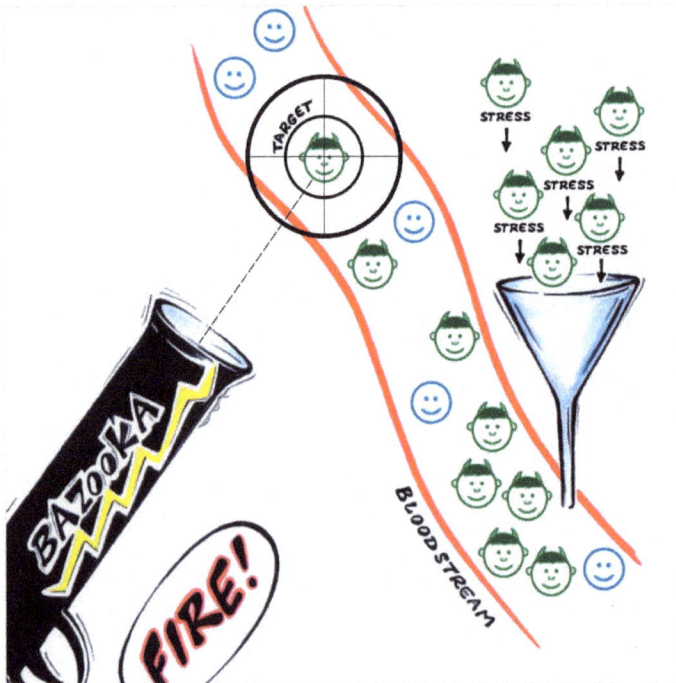

The first person I interviewed who reversed her cancer without any treatments or supplements was Kleri, a woman in her 40s from Hamilton, Ontario, Canada. After a lump was found in her right breast, she realized that the relationship challenge she had with her partner had pushed her body past its limit. She was told by her oncologist that she would have to go to war on her cancer, and an appointment was scheduled for treatments. Kleri had over a month to wait for the treatment, and so, she decided to get away from all the stress and lack of fulfilment in her life, which included a decision to separate from her partner.

She travelled to British Columbia, Canada, and spent a month in nature while she learned how to surf. She cried a lot during that trip, while she was alone walking in the majestic old-growth forests of BC. Connecting to her heart, processing and ultimately accepting the pain of her past, her current reality, and her fear of the future, she began healing. She was determined to create a new life that would bring her real happiness. Each day she felt lighter and more independent.

When she arrived back in Ontario and went to her oncologist, she was assessed again and the tumour in her breast was gone. Her oncologist said "we must have made a mistake when we initially tested you". Kleri, however, knew what happened – **she healed herself from within.** Facing her fears, shedding emotional pain and judgment, and energizing a new dream, transformed her life, and her body.

> *By not focusing on the root cause of cancer, but instead focusing on destroying cancer, a battle begins that often ends tragically.*

Currently, traditional treatments are considered successful when cancer cells are no longer diagnostically measurable. But, current technology cannot find cancer cells in our body unless they have accumulated to a size larger than the diameter of a pencil lead (which is still approximately one million cancer cells in size!).[97] In other words, even when deemed "cancer-free" after treatments, there may still be millions of cancer cells in a person's body.

Consider the words of Dr Thomas Lodi (fellow speaker at the Cure to Cancer Conference in San Diego, 2014):

> *"It doesn't matter how good anyone is at getting rid of cancer – if you're still producing cancer, it will be back. Any program that does not include how to stop producing cancer cells should automatically be suspect – of course it is not going to be effective."[98]*

The glucose-absorbing quality of cancer cells has been known for a long time. In the early 1900s, Nobel Prize-winning doctor, Otto Warburg may have been the first person to discover the connection between glucose and cancer cells. This connection was termed the "Warburg Effect", and in his book, *The Prime Cause and Prevention of Cancer*, he wrote:

> *"Cancer, above all other diseases, has countless secondary causes, but there is only one prime cause... the replacement of the normal oxygen respiration of body cells by anaerobic cell respiration [glucose metabolism]."[99]*

Anaerobic glycolysis is the process that takes place in cancer cells whereby glucose is metabolized. One of the byproducts of this process is lactic acid.[100] This is why in later stages of cancer, fluid begins to build in the body and can become extremely uncomfortable and painful.

It is normal for the cells of our body to absorb glucose for energy. However, cancer cells are unique – they absorb far more glucose than normal. Do cancer cells protect our body by soaking up the otherwise damaging effects of excess localized blood glucose? Do chronic surges in glucose trigger the growth of cancer cells? And do continued surges provide them with fuel? **Cancer cells may be an effort by our body to protect itself from the damaging effects of excess glucose – the result of stress and dietary factors in our life.**

Today, researchers are beginning to see the significant interdependence between glucose and cancer. Don Ayer, PhD, Professor of the Department of Oncological Sciences at the University of Utah, states the following: **"It has been known since 1923 that tumour cells use a lot more glucose than normal cells.**[101] Ayer discovered that when the availability of glucose is restricted, cancer cells cannot continue to grow. According to Ayer, "The cancer cell is short-circuited due to a lack of glucose, which halts the growth of the tumour."[102]

Throughout the body, the glucose consumption rate of various types of cells: for example, brain cells are some of the highest consumers of blood glucose. Yet, cancer cells still absorb about twice as much glucose than brain cells.[103]

For any cell in our body to absorb glucose from the bloodstream, it requires insulin receptors. The more insulin receptors a cell has, the more capable it is of absorbing glucose. **Compared to normal cells, cancer cells have 23 times more insulin receptors, making them exceptionally good at absorbing glucose.** [104]

One of the ways oncologists diagnose cancer is by measuring a patient's Standardized Sugar Uptake Value, by injecting radioactive sugar into their bloodstream. If cancer cells are present, they will absorb much more of that sugar than regular cells out

BLOODSTREAM

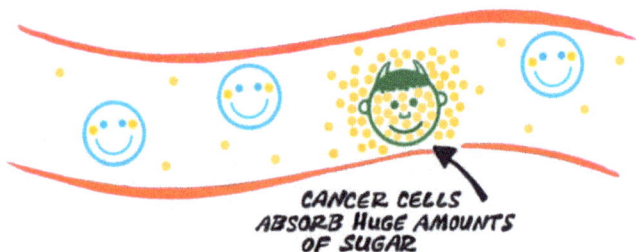

CANCER CELLS
ABSORB HUGE AMOUNTS
OF SUGAR

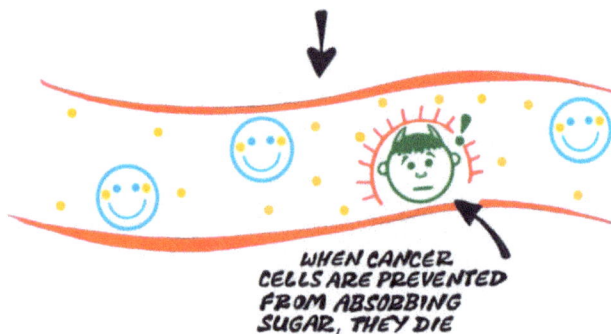

WHEN CANCER
CELLS ARE PREVENTED
FROM ABSORBING
SUGAR, THEY DIE

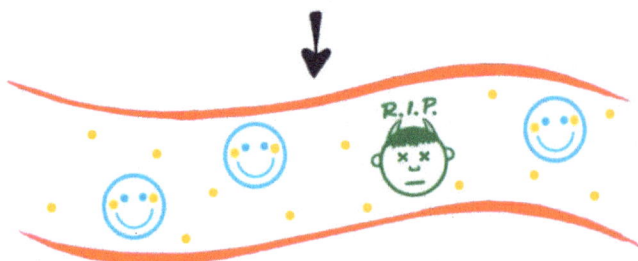

of the bloodstream, revealing their location in a PET scan.[105]

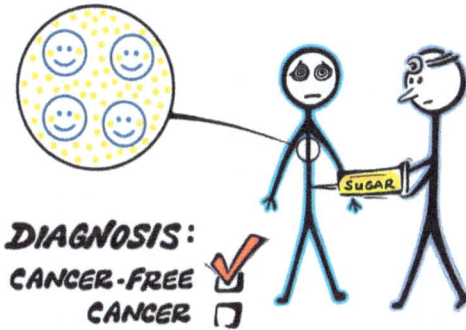

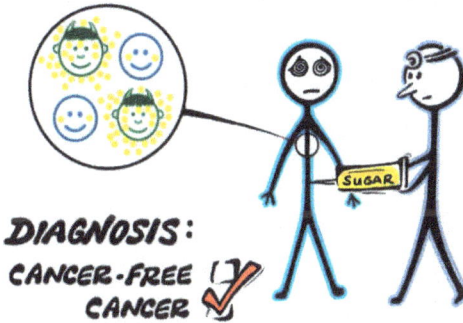

I'm sure you've heard of lung, colon, breast, pancreas, and liver cancer. But, how often do you hear of heart cancer? The heart is a muscle that uses glucose as fuel, 24 hours a day; it is the only muscle in the body that never stops contracting. As a result, the heart is much less prone to the damaging effects of excess glucose. Additionally, each time the Stress Response initiates, it stimulates the heart to beat faster, which increases its consumption of glucose. Heart cancer is so rare, that it accounts for less than 0.01% of all cancers.[106]

Recall from chapter 3 that our immune system does not attack cancer cells. The reason may not be that it can't recognize cancer cells or is not strong enough to battle against them, but that **cancer cells have a purpose in our body; they absorb excess blood glucose.** Just like the various survival-responses mentioned, cancer also has its associated drawbacks, and indeed, if what's fueling cancer's growth is not addressed, cancer will destroy our body. **Perhaps our immune system only eliminates cancer cells when they no longer serve a purpose.** This is what happens in spontaneous remissions, where a person's cancer vanishes without undergoing any treatments or attempts to destroy it.

Cancer cells only show up when an individual has entered into a survival state. It is their body mirroring back to them that something in their life needs to change. Cancer appears for a meaningful reason, not because of a cellular error.

The real reason for a spontaneous remission is that a person has experienced significant, positive change, and their motivation for life has been renewed. This resolves the factors that cause excess blood glucose, and therefore their cancer. For the 50% of people who undergo treatments and survive beyond the 5-year mark, **the real reason why cancer did not grow back is likely because the individual simultaneously changed their life and inadvertently addressed the root cause of their cancer.**

ROOT CAUSE PRACTITIONER TRAINING

I just wanted to thank you and your team for such a wonderful experience throughout the course. I have learned so much and I can't wait to bring the knowledge you have shared with us to my clients.
-Christina

This course was incredible! Thank you so much for bringing this to us and to the world!
-Lyndsay

Having recently finished Root Cause Practitioner training with Paul, I can wholeheartedly recommend this course to anyone looking for guidance and support, either for their own self healing or for deepening their capacity to support other peoples' healing journeys.

It was deeply moving and encouraging for me on multiple levels and it felt truly magical to experience Paul's work.

As a teacher, Paul shares his wisdom with a depth of courage and humility which is rare to find in our world today and hearing the insight with which he tells his own personal stories and the stories of his clients, without drama or ego, is both inspiring and refreshing. Thank you Paul!
-Samantha

Thank you for the experience and sharing your knowledge. This was a truly wonderful and well invested program.
-Dianna

8

100 POUNDS OF POISON

Refined sugar is one of the most ubiquitous food substances eaten today, and is likely a major contributing factor in the growth of cancer cells. Refined sugar is often hidden in processed foods and comes in many inconspicuous forms. Most people have no idea just how much refined sugar they are consuming.

If you recall the damage that high blood glucose does to the body (chapter 5), you may not be surprised to know that **refined sugar, by definition, is a poison.** According to Encyclopedia Britannica, a poison is: "Any substance, natural or synthetic, that causes damage to living tissues and has an injurious or fatal effect on the body, whether ingested, inhaled, absorbed or injected through the skin."[107]

Not only does refined sugar harm our bodies, but it is extremely addictive. Alcohol, cigarettes, and coffee are known for their addictive natures, but many people have no idea that **refined sugar is one of the most addictive substances on the planet.** If you have not yet already done so, try cutting it out of your diet and see for yourself!

Another common addiction is caffeine, which is a drug that causes a Stress-Response in the body when ingested. Research shows that caffeine increases the stress hormone cortisol[108], which causes blood glucose surges.

Thus, both caffeine and refined sugar commonly cause an artificial "boost of energy" or temporary uplifting of emotions when consumed. This is important to understand because, often, when individuals cut out refined sugar, they begin consuming more caffeine to make up for the "loss of energy", and drop in emotions, and vice versa. Actually, over time, my observations have shown me that **both refined sugar and caffeine slowly drain energy from our body, bring our emotions down, leading to a downward spiral, that is difficult to break since both are addictive.**

The challenge then is to substantially **reduce and, if possible, eliminate both of them from your diet** (which is not an easy task). If you can accomplish this, you will notice after a few weeks that you're overall feeling of vitality, healthy emotions, and energy will have risen substantially. Your mind will also likely become more clear, with better memory. Additionally, you'll likely lose some excess weight, if you haver any. With regards to cancer, it is highly supportive to cut out both refined sugar and caffeine, because both of them lead to blood glucose surges which feed cancer cells.

A very good book on the damaging effects of refined sugar is "Sugar Blues" by William Dufty, and a good book on the damaging effects of caffeine is "Caffeine Blues" by Stephen Cherniske. Together, these two books can change your life if you have either of these addictions and suffer from the symptoms they can cause (chronic pain, excess weight, depression, dysbiosis – a disruption in the microbiome of our gut – the list goes on and on.)

NOTE: I am currently creating a course on how to overcome addictions such as these. If you need help, please look on my website to see if it's available yet (www.rootcauseinstitute.com). If it

is not, subscribe to my emails at the bottom of any page of the website to be notified when it's ready, along with other helpful resources and courses I am continually creating.

Below is an excerpt from William Dufty's "Sugar Blues", which illustrates a striking parallel between sugar and opiates:

> *"After all, heroin is nothing but a chemical. They take the juice of the poppy and they refine it into opium and then they refine it to morphine and finally to heroin. Sugar is nothing but a chemical. They take the juice of the cane or the beet, and they refine it to molasses and then they refine it to brown sugar and finally to strange white crystals. It's no wonder dope pushers dilute pure heroin with milk sugar (lactose) to make their glassine packages a treat to the eye."[109]*

Research on refined sugar from world-famous Neuroscientist, Candace Pert, author of "Molecules of Emotion", concluded her suggesting refined sugar be classified as a "Class 1 Drug, equally as dangerous as heroine."[110]

Dr John Briffa, one of Britain's foremost experts in the field of complementary medicine states that "one teaspoon of refined sugar can suppress the immune system for several hours."[111] Knowing this, consider the fact that there are up to 10 teaspoons of refined sugar in just one can of pop, and every single day, The Coca-Cola Company alone sells over 1.7 billion cans.[112]

In the past, human beings consumed only nutrient-dense whole foods; Food did not need to be labeled as "certified organic" because it was already grown organically by Mother Nature. Today, many foods have become dangerous – commonly sprayed with pesticides and other toxic chemicals; highly processed, or are not really food at all.

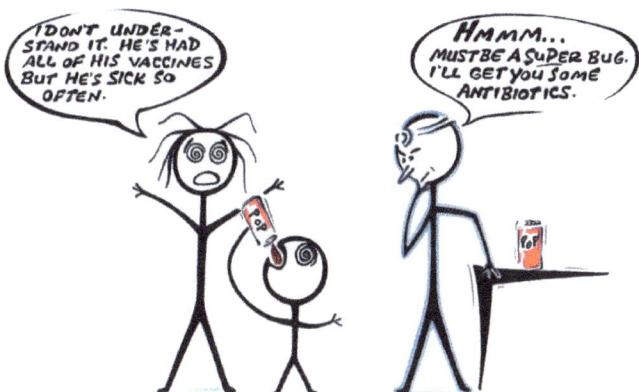

In 1700 the average person in America ate around 4 pounds of refined sugar per year; in 1900, 60 pounds per year; and as of 2012 that number had skyrocketed to **over 100 pounds per year, per person.**[113] The rare person exists who does not eat refined sugar, but for every person who does not eat refined sugar, it means someone else could be eating 200 pounds per year.

TIP

If you want to stop eating refined sugar, an effective strategy is to fulfill sugar cravings from real food. All fruits are healthy, but some are especially low in sugar (important if you have cancer), such as blueberries, strawberries, blackberries, raspberries, green apples and grapefruit. If you have cancer, keep to a minimum high glycemic fruits like bananas, mangoes, and grapes, for example. Practice saying no to refined sugar when offered by friends and family. Remember not to force or pressure your new values on anyone.

1900

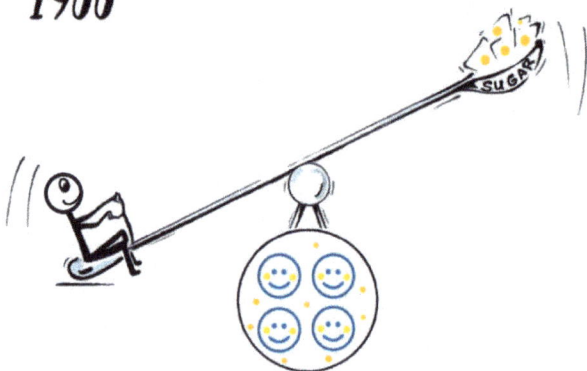

2012

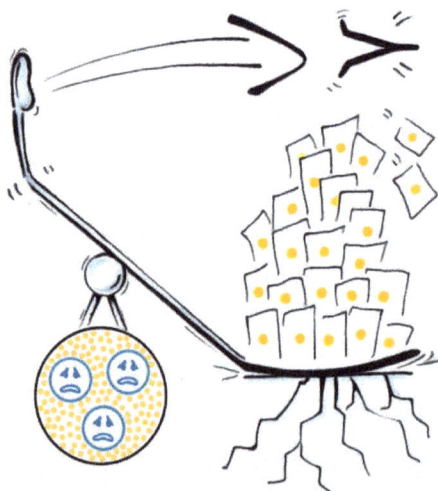

Would it be too much to say that refined sugar has become a threat to the well-being of the entire human race? For example, Type II Diabetes was rare in 1900 but has increased 30-fold in the last 15 years,[114] and in that same period the rate of cancer has risen 1500%.[115]

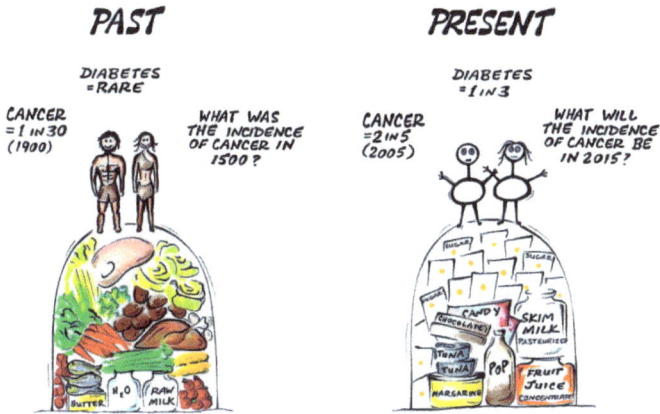

PAST

CANCER = 1 IN 30 (1900)

DIABETES = RARE

WHAT WAS THE INCIDENCE OF CANCER IN 1500?

BUTTER H_2O RAW MILK

PRESENT

CANCER = 2 IN 5 (2005)

DIABETES = 1 IN 3

WHAT WILL THE INCIDENCE OF CANCER BE IN 2015?

SUGAR SUGAR CANDY CHOCOLATE SKIM MILK PASTEURIZED TUNA POP MARGARINE FRUIT JUICE CONCENTRATE

Refined sugar has been extracted and isolated from natural, whole foods. Isolating components of food alters the way they interact with our body, compromising our health in some way or another. After we eat food, its nutrition and life-energy is absorbed into our body; Food is first broken down and digested by our mouth and stomach, and then it's absorbed into our bloodstream. What's not useful is excreted.

The process of digestion, assimilation, and elimination requires our body's energy and nutrition. Refined sugar is classified as an "anti-nutrient" because after its ingestion, while it may give a quick boost of energy or pleasure, it also causes damage in the many ways already mentioned. Overall, our body loses more nutrients and energy than it gains from refined sugar (far more).[116] Conversely, **organic whole foods provide more energy and nutrients than they take to be processed by our body – this is why after an organic whole food meal, people generally feel more light, awake, happy, and energized, with no side effects.**

Organic whole foods always contain a variety of nutrients bound together with their inherent sugar; this causes the sugar molecules contained in the food to gradually absorb into the bloodstream, allowing the pancreas (which produces insulin) to easily manage the incoming sugar, maintaining homeostasis.

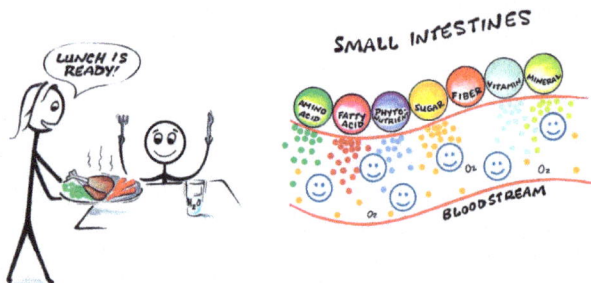

For our body to remain in a healthy state of homeostasis, it must also maintain blood pH levels. If pH gets either too low (acidosis) or too high (alkalosis), it is life-threatening, just as with all other variables in our bloodstream which must remain balanced.[117]

Ingesting refined sugar causes our bloodstream to become acidic, forcing our body into yet another energy-and-resource-consuming survival response: our body must break down its own tissue (including teeth and bones) to access calcium, which has an alkalizing effect on the bloodstream. This helps to counterbalance the acidity caused by refined sugar.[118]

SMALL INTESTINES

BLOODSTREAM

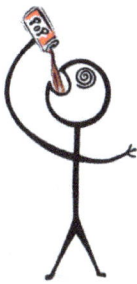

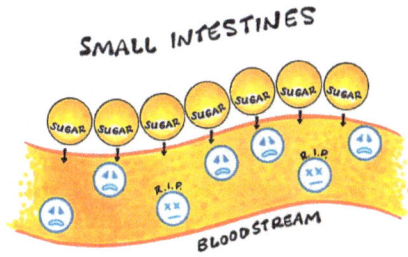

If you drink coffee, you'll notice soon afterwards, the need to urinate. Research shows that large quantities of calcium are lost in urine soon after ingesting caffeine.[119] Caffeine also causes the blood to become acidic, which leaches calcium from bones and teeth. Long time coffee drinkers often have cavities or holes in their teeth as a result, and weaker bones. Osteoporosis is a very common disease around the world, for example 3 million people are afflicted in the United Kingdom, 2.3 million people in Canada, and 1.2 million people in Australia.[120]

JAYNE'S CANCER REVERSAL

I was diagnosed with breast cancer and told that I would need a full mastectomy and lymph nodes removed. After the initial shock wore off, I got a second opinion and was offered a much less radical option of a lumpectomy. Although that was a better option it still didn't feel like the right choice for me, especially given that they also wanted to do radiation, and likely chemo. I decided to do my best to heal without surgery or chemicals and I booked my stay with Paul Leendertse.

What a life-changing experience. It was so peaceful there and the meals that were so lovingly prepared were exceptional. Aside from the lovely getaway, the time spent in nature, and the awesome time making music, what I valued most was the incredible amount of one on one time that Paul spent with me, teaching me so much and giving such good council. I came away with a clear understanding of what I needed to do to get well, and I'm healing my cancer now, from within. I feel so blessed to have had the opportunity to work with Paul.

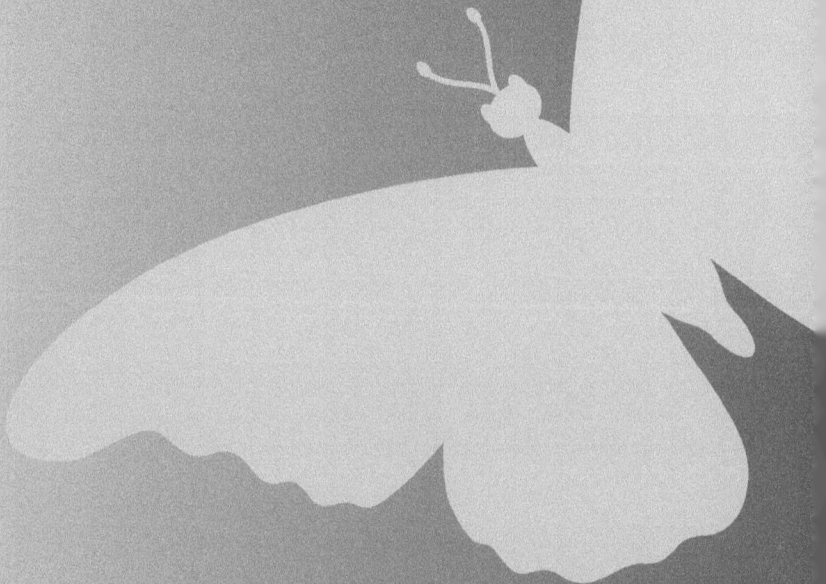

9

POISON DISGUISED

Recall that cancer cells have been proven to stop growing when they lose access to sugar, and additionally, cancer cells have been proven to multiply in response to more sugar. Therefore, it is in the best interest of everyone, whether diagnosed with cancer or not, to avoid refined sugar.

Avoiding refined sugar may sound easy – all you have to do is stop scooping sugar out of the sugar bowl, right? That is essential but there's more to be aware of. In "How to Eat, Move and Be Healthy!", Paul Chek lists important facts for identifying refined sugar which may be lurking in the foods you are purchasing:

- The order of the ingredients listed on a food product represents the proportion of weight from highest to lowest. In other words, **the first ingredient on the list makes up the majority of the food product.** If you pay attention to this while you shop for food, you'll notice refined sugar is at the top of the list of many foods.

- Ingredients that end with "ose" are refined sugar. Examples are fructose (refined from fruit), lactose (refined from milk), maltose (refined from barley), and so on. In particular, be aware of fructose and "high-fructose corn syrup"; research published in 2010 by the American Association for Cancer Research concluded that fructose, without a doubt, promotes pancreatic cancer growth.[122]

- Some other sneaky words that are simply refined sugar are maltodextrin, malt syrup, invert sugar, corn syrup solids, molasses, fruit juice concentrate, cane crystals, evaporated cane juice or syrup, and many more.[123]

One more to look out for is "agave syrup", which is commonly advertised as a healthy sweetener, but contains very high levels of fructose and very few nutrients. Since large food corporations develop and market new forms of refined sugar and sugar-substitutes regularly, **I strongly suggest eating whole foods only – which simply have no ingredient list!**

TIP

Unpasteurized raw honey (used sparingly: 1–2 teaspoons a day) is one of the healthiest and safest sweeteners. Not surprisingly, it is made from Nature (bees). The next best option may be maple syrup, since it also provided by Nature (trees) – but it still goes through a refinement process which increases its sugar content (and sometimes involves chemicals).

NOTE: Pesticides used in commercial farming kill bees. I happen to live beside a large non-organic orchard that is sprayed with poison each year, and each time I watch countless bees drop dead on my front porch. It hurts my heart to have to witness this...

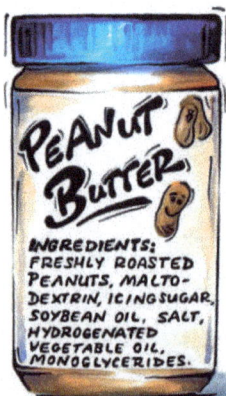

Let's look at an example of the ingredient list in a common processed food: peanut butter. Peanut butter should be made of peanuts right? This peanut butter example does contain some peanuts (32%). It also contains refined sugar in the form of maltodextrin (29%) and icing sugar (29%), which together make up over half the contents of the "peanut butter". And it contains soybean oil (3%), salt (3%), hydrogenated vegetable oil (2%) and monoglycerides (2%). It would make more sense to call it a "refined-sugar product with peanuts".

TIP
Some food manufacturers avoid using refined sugar (and chemicals) in their products. Now that you know how to identify refined sugar on ingredient lists, you can spend your money wisely by supporting businesses who have integrity and care about your health.

Other High Glucose Foods
To protect your body from glucose damage, you need to be aware of 3 additional processed foods. They are:

- Pasteurized milk
- Pasteurized juice from concentrate
- Flour

Pasteurized Milk
Pasteurization is a food processing technique that uses a high temperature treatment or boiling process that destroys the life-force of milk and other liquids to "reduce pathogens" and increase shelf life. Ultra-pasteurized milk, for example, involves heating milk far over boiling point, to at least 138 C, which increases the shelf life of milk to up to 3 months.[124] Whereas, healthy raw milk lasts only about a week.

I grew up on a farm, and we knew as farmers, that **if we fed our calves pasteurized milk, they would get sick and likely die.** Only raw milk will keep a calf alive and well, this is because, as I have said, pasteurized milk is dead – it has no more life-force energy. Essentially, life-force energy is what leaves a person's body when they die. On a heart monitor this is seen as a flat-line. The foods which are most supportive of our body are foods that contain high amounts of life-force. Refined sugar does not contain any life-force. This is why refined sugar also has an extremely long shelf-life (it is dead, like pasteurized milk), but fruit, which contains life-force, goes bad within days or weeks after being picked (it dies); and very quickly, once it's cut open.

Pasteurization of milk destroys its valuable nutrients, including Vitamin B12, Vitamin C, all of its enzymes (which are essential for digestion – including lactase, the enzyme that digests lactose), and more.[125] However, pasteurization does not destroy the sugar, which results in milk with a higher-than-normal sugar content. Often, factories that process milk also remove part or most of its fat, creating low fat milk, or "skim milk": Raw, nutrient-dense milk is turned into a refined-sugar-laden liquid that is low in nutrients, which can flood your bloodstream with glucose.

TIP
To fulfill your body's need for calcium (and many other nutrients), you can eat organic green vegetables and make your own bone broths. For those who do well with dairy, just ensure any milk you consume is raw and from pasture-raised animals.

While I do suggest cutting out all pasteurized milk (including homogenized), I do not suggest cutting out organic butter. This might be surprising for some because of fear of cholesterol. On this topic, I suggest reading "The Great Cholesterol Myth", by Jimmy Moore and especially Nourishing Traditions, by Sally Fallon.

In summary, cholesterol is actually one of the most essential building blocks of hormones in our body, the carrier of important fat-soluble vitamins, and more. Breast milk, for example, contains high levels of cholesterol for growing babies, and our liver naturally manufacture's cholesterol because it is so important for health.[126]

Pasteurized Juice

The damaging effects of pasteurization also apply to fruit and vegetables – if you drink pasteurized juice (or juice from concentrate), it's very similar to drinking refined sugar. It is wise to drink only freshly pressed juice, ideally immediately after juicing it. You'll notice that freshly pressed juice begins to turn brown very quickly – this is due to oxidation and the loss of life-force energy. NOTE: Although juicing provides beneficial nutrients which are easily absorbed, it also delivers a higher than normal amount of sugar compared to eating fruit or vegetables in their whole form.

NOTE: Even though juicing is a part of many popular cancer protocols, it's something I only suggest to my clients under rare, unique circumstances. Our body is designed for consistent whole food meals, which most optimally fulfills our nutritional, energetic, and regenerative needs.

TIP

Clean water is one of the most important liquids to drink to support the prevention or reversal of cancer. The average person can only survive for about 3 days without consuming water, before dying of dehydration. If you are not hydrated, it does not matter how good any supplement, "cure", or "treatment" for cancer may be. As a general rule, **it is essential to drink half your body weight in ounces of water each day.**[127]

The best water is uncontaminated spring water or well water, but as the Earth is becoming more and more polluted, almost all natural sources of water are contaminated to some degree. Today, a variety of filtration systems exist for removing the many contaminants from the environment and those commonly added to water (such as chlorine, flouride, arsenic, and more). There are activated carbon filters (such as Berkey) that do not remove the natural minerals from your water, but significantly reduce contaminants. NOTE: The Berkey is not ideal for removing arsenic and flouride. Another popular filtration system is reverse osmosis which removes far greater amounts of pollutants, but also depletes the water of its natural minerals. So if you use reverse osmosis, it's important to add minerals back to your water; an easy way to do this is by adding a pinch of unrefined sea salt to your water (not so much that you can taste it).

There are far more options available for water filtration. To optimize the water you drink and bathe in, the best approach is to first get your water tested, to see what contaminants you need to filter, and then find an appropriate filter.

Drink from glass or stainless steel bottles as much as possible, and avoid plastic, which contaminates your body and our planet.

White Flour

Last in this list of foods to avoid is white flour. According to David Getoff, Vice President of the Price-Pottenger Foundation, the way most grains are grown and processed today makes consuming them detrimental to our body for various reasons:[128]

1. Grains have been extensively hybridized and are often genetically modified, which alone can cause stress to our body. According to the Center For Food Safety, **genetically modified foods have been scientifically proven to have the**

following health risks (associations): toxicity, allergic reactions, antibiotic resistance, immuno-suppression, cancer (breast, prostate and colon), and loss of nutrition.[129]

2. Secondly, refining grains into white flour, removes the bran and the germ, resulting in a refined carbohydrate-rich food. Refined carbohydrates are sugar molecules linked together which quickly turn into blood glucose after consumption.

3. Grinding grains into flour increases their surface area by many thousands of times. The surface area of the intestines is where nutrients are absorbed into our bloodstream. This area is enormous – the size of a tennis court.[130] The finely ground particles of flour coat a very large surface area of the intestinal wall, which quickly absorbs the carbohydrate-rich food, causing a blood glucose surge. The following analogy is helpful: Imagine covering a tennis court with eggs placed side by side. Only a tiny portion of each egg (the bottom tip) would make contact with the surface of the court. But if the eggs were crushed into powder, they would make contact with the entire surface area at once.

4. Gluten is found in most grains and has been shown to cause permanent damage to the intestines due to chronic inflammation. According to Dr Bill Timmins, ND, Founder of Biohealth Diagnostics in San Diego, over 60% of caucasians are gluten intolerant[131] and 99% of them are unaware.[132] The following symptoms can be caused by eating gluten.[133] If you are not officially gluten intolerant, you may still benefit from eliminating gluten from your diet.

• Abdominal pain and cramping or distensions (beer belly)
• Alternating bouts of diarrhea and constipation
• Anemia
• Arthritis

- Asthma
- Attention Deficit Disorder
- Autism
- Back pain, and bloating
- Bone density loss
- Borborygmi
- Cramps
- Stunted growth
- Depression, anxiety and irritability
- Dermatitis herpetiformis
- Diabetes
- Eczema
- Fatigue
- Headache
- Joint pain
- Foul-smelling flatulence and stools
- Menstrual cycle pain
- Miscarriage
- Nutritional deficiencies due to mal-absorption eg. Low Iron
- Gluten ataxia
- Greyish stools
- Hair loss, headaches and migraines
- Infertility
- Juvenile idiopathic arthritis
- Lactose intolerance
- Mouth sores or mouth ulcers
- Nausea
- Numbness or tingling in the hands and feet
- Osteoporosis
- Peripheral neuropathy
- Sjorgen's disease
- Steatorrhea teeth and gum problems
- Turner syndrome
- Vitamin and mineral deficiencies

- Vomiting
- Unexplained weight loss
- Urinary tract infections
- Urticaria

Paul Chek, founder of the CHEK Institute suggests an effective way to determine if you are gluten intolerant: Remove all sources of grains (bread, doughnuts, pasta, etc) from your diet for one month. After 30 days, eat gluten again and see what happens to your body.[134]

TIP
To prevent or reverse cancer (especially in any part of the digestive tract), remove all sources of white flour and gluten-containing grains from your diet. If you have cancer, I suggest eliminating all grains from your diet, and eating only life-force rich, whole foods.

While it may seem overwhelming to somehow avoid so many sources of refined sugar and other high-blood-glucose-causing foods, the solution is actually simple: Make a goal to consistently eat home-made meals comprised of whole foods, and drink water. Focus on discovering and enjoying all the various real foods that exist (there are many!).

▶ **Suggested Videos**
PricePottenger Presents: Mark McAfee and the Raw Milk Secret
www.youtube.com/watch?v=9BILdZDB-XoSugar: The Bitter Truth
www.youtube.com/watch?v=dBnniua6-oM

📖 **Suggested Books**
Sugar Blues, by William Dufty
Caffeine Blues, by Stephen Cherniske

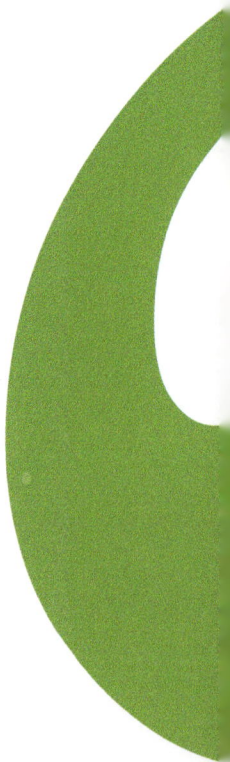

ROOT CAUSE COACHING

Hi Paul, thank you again for a profoundly moving and life changing coaching session!

Lynda wanted me to tell you really got her! She took my notes with her to use in her alone time on her commute.
We are truly GRATEFUL to you!

The oncologist's nurse called her a short while ago regarding the scan and said "Nothing to worry about", (!) Thank you again.
Blessings,
Jim and Lynda

10

FOOD AND "FOOD"

There's more to know about processed foods beyond their direct blood-glucose elevating effects – they also contain seriously damaging compounds that add physical stress to our bodies. **Scientists have discovered that when they feed laboratory animals the same ingredients found in common processed foods, the animals frequently develop cancer.**[135] How many people are aware that they are purchasing and eating scientifically proven carcinogens on a daily basis?

The nutrients we ingest in our food are the building blocks of our body. Just like a car requires many different parts to perform properly, each human cell requires all sorts of working parts to function optimally, and those parts come from our food. While the different parts of a car are built separately and then assembled into a working vehicle, different food components in our diet are built by nature, we eat them, and then our body assembles them into a living vehicle.[136]

The human body replaces itself constantly. About once per year, 98% of its cells are manufactured anew.[137] The liver is entirely replaced every 6 weeks; the skin every 4 weeks, and our skeleton in just three months.[138] The body is a master of maintenance and regeneration – provided it gets all it needs from us, the operator. An important question is: what are you building your body out of – a mixture of chemicals, or real food?

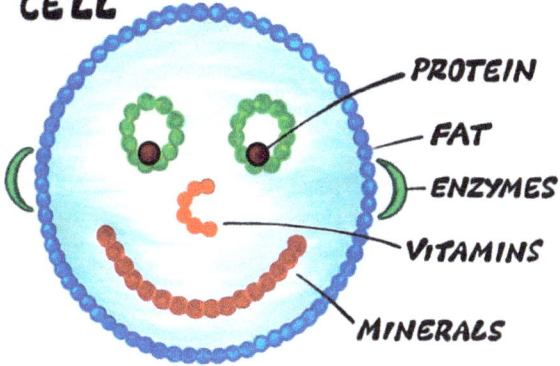

HUMAN CELL

PROTEIN
FAT
ENZYMES
VITAMINS
MINERALS

In "A Shopper's Guide to What's Safe and What's Not", Christine Farlow estimates that the average American consumes approximately 150 pounds of food additives per year.[139] For some people, that might be more than their body weight.

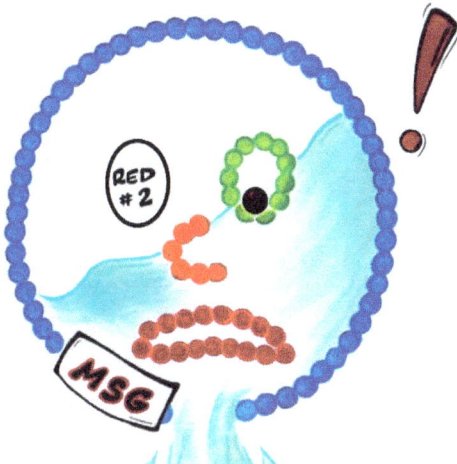

RED #2

MSG

If our body is forced to attempt to build itself out of processed foods (additives, preservatives, "natural" flavour, coloring agents, emulsifiers, monosodium glutamate, refined sugar, gluten, and poor quality fats and proteins) **it will eventually fail, and be compromised all along the way; because it cannot build itself properly out of non-foods.**

Our immune and detoxification systems can remove toxins that enter our body, but these systems have limits. If too many toxins overwhelm our body, our organs become worn out and inflamed. In "Beating the Food Giants", Paul Stitt writes:

> *"Processed foods are terrible things for our body for two reasons – they are stripped of their nutrient value in the refining process, and they are poisoned with refined sugar and other harmful additives."[140]*

One must wonder, "what is the true intention of a company which adds harmful substances to food"?

In the past, food was actually food, but today we have three distinct types of "food" to choose from: artificial "food", non-organic (commercially farmed) "food", and finally, real food.

1. Artificial Food
These are corporation-made, processed foods containing a long list of chemicals. The law states that any manufactured "food" must display at least a partial list of ingredients.

STORY

When I was in my 20's, I learned about artificial food and realized that my fridge and cupboards were full of them. I also realized that my back pain at the time, skin problems, and my inability to sleep through the night were a result of essentially poisoning myself with "food" that I assumed was safe, and normal to consume. My partner and I went through our fridge and all our cupboards, and threw everything out that wasn't pure food; 2 garbage bags worth of artificial non-foods.

From that point on, the quality of every aspect of our life improved; our energy levels increased, symptoms in our body disappeared, our connection with each other deepened, our productivity rose, and emotional well-being heightened.

2. Commercially Farmed Food (real food, yet laced with poisons)

Though technically a real food, non-organic produce is contaminated with pesticides, herbicides, and other chemicals that poison our bodies, as well as the soil, water and air of our planet. Fruits and vegetables may also be genetically modified or irradiated, neither of which have any long-term studies that demonstrate their safety, **but have been correlated with breast, prostate and colon cancer.**[141] Commercially-farmed meat is toxic: animals are confined inside buildings with little or no windows, fed formulated diets designed to fatten them as quickly as possible without any real regard for their health. Not surprisingly, they are often sick and die prematurely; heavily medicated with pharmaceutical drugs, antibiotics, steroids, and vaccines. Many have disease at the time of slaughter.

Once you realize what's happening in the case of many countries such as Canada and the United States, it may dawn on you that you don't generally see any real farm animals out in the country-side. You can buy bacon in the grocery stores, but where are all the pigs? You can buy chicken in the grocery stores, but where are all the chickens? The next time you go for a drive in the country side, see if you can find all the hidden, window-less, buildings often built far back from the road – those buildings are full of disease-ridden animals which supply the shelves of most grocery stores with meat. What has happened to the consciousness of the human race?

STORY

When I was younger I owned a construction business. One year when I laid off my foreman during the off-season winter months, he worked in a commercial turkey factory for some supplementary income. His job was to collect all the dead turkeys that appeared daily on the cement floor. He told me that each day, he would walk through the hundreds of birds all crammed together in that dark building, and carry out 20–40 dead ones. Every day, the same reality. The birds lived in their own feces, had no fresh air or sunlight, were crowded together, and stood and slept on a concrete floor. A pharmaceutical representative would come once per week and add drugs to the water-supply of the chickens, and all the birds would be vaccinated. The flock started with 4000 baby turkeys and ended with a few hundred, the rest all having died of disease. The remaining living turkeys were then packed into a truck and shipped off to a slaughter house, and finally to a grocery store.

They are then purchased mostly by people who have either no idea what they are supporting with their dollars, do not care, want to save money, or do not know how toxic this meat is and how it was raised.

3. Holistic-farmed, Organic Whole foods (Real, love-based food)

Fruits and vegetables are grown from healthy soil, clean water, sunlight, and the loving intentions of the farmers. They do not use artificial fertilizers or pesticides, so this food is clean. Animalsare raised happily and lovingly, outside on pasture; they absorb sunlight, breathe fresh clean air, and can run and play. With the case of turkeys or chickens, they are also outside foraging, and if needed, are supplemented with organic grains. By no surprise, **these animals are exceptionally healthy (and happy) without drugs, antibiotics, or vaccines, and rarely need medical intervention of any kind.**[142]

In book 2, I will talk more about eating meat, emotional pain, and accepting death as part of life. What certainly is not acceptable is disrespecting the life-experience of an animal, and raising it for profit-only, inhumanely. A very good book on raising your own food is "The Self-Sufficient Life and How to Live it", by John Seymore. This book has rare knowledge about animal husbandry and growing organic food consciously.

NOTE: I have spoken at several cancer symposiums and worldwide cancer conventions, and here is what I observed: scientists are running experiments to study the benefits or detriments of eating meat, particularly associated with cancer. All studies I have seen presented, have been done on commercially-raised (unhealthy!) animals, or the scientists "didn't know" how the animals were raised, when I asked them. This kind of "science" is like studying the effects of drinking polluted water, and then drawing the conclusion (and publishing the results!) that water is not healthy to drink. This is not valuable science.

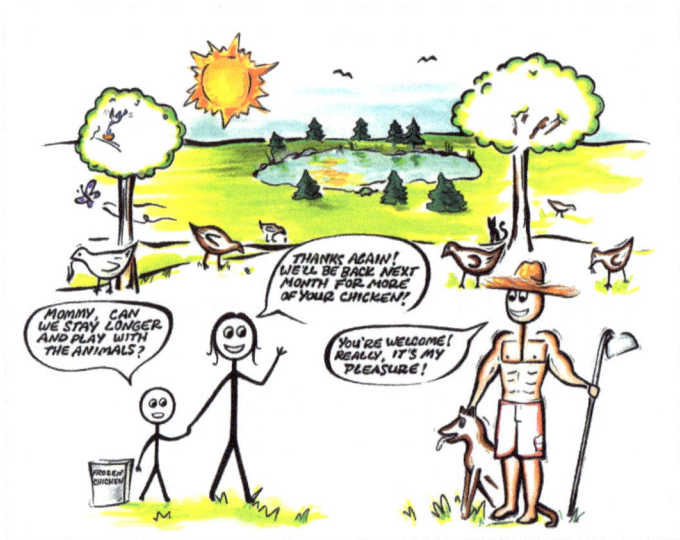

I suggest never eating meat unless you know for sure that it comes from a loving, conscious farmer, and this usually requires searching for and personally meeting the farmer and observing what kind of life they are providing for their animals. If the meat is raised with love, it will be full of nutrition and good energy, from an animal that lived a beautiful, sheltered, cared-for life.

STORY
I have personally raised my own food. I normally have sheep, goats, chickens, ducks, geese, rabbits, and sometimes a cow. All of my animals live together and share plenty of forest and pasture-space. They play, they relax in the shade, tan in the sun, and emanate happiness every day of their lives. They are like a big happy family. I have not had a single animal die of disease in my entire life as a hobby farmer.

All sorts of chemicals in food have supposedly been "scientifically proven to be safe for consumption". However, most studies done on the effects of processed food are only short-term studies,[143] and are carried out by none other than the food manufacturers themselves! Muti-billion dollar corporations can afford to plan, design, and carry out their "research" trials to justify what they sell is "safe for consumption."

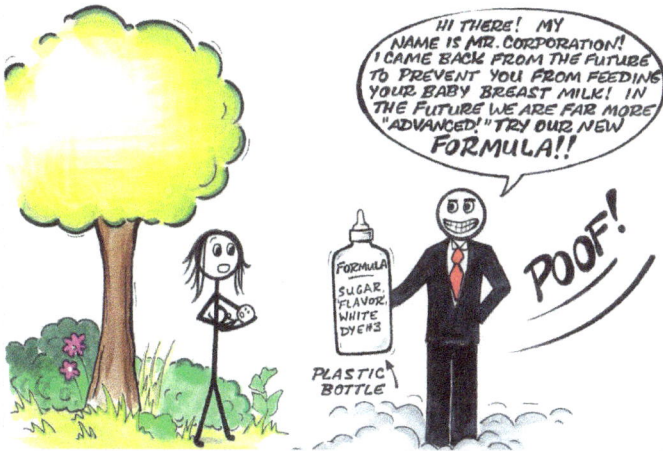

Most large corporations spend more money on advertising than they do on the quality of the products they sell. Children are often the main targets for processed food ads because they are too young and trusting to think for themselves. If you tell a child that processed foods are safe to eat, and you provide them with these foods, most will eat them. In a recent survey in Australia, nine and ten-year-old children were asked if Ronald McDonald knew more about nutrition than their mother. It turns out 50% of those children believed that Ronald McDonald knows better.[145] It should come as no surprise that childhood cancer is the leading cause of disease-related death among children in the United States, and rates are increasing by approximately 1% each year.[146]

According to the Food and Drug Administration of America (FDA), some children eat as much as a quarter-pound of food colouring per year.[147] The food colours listed below have been banned from being added to food, after it was discovered they were associated with cancer and other major health issues.[148]

FD&C Violet #1
FD&C Red #2
D&C Red #10-13
D&C Yellow #1

TIP
By focusing on providing yourself and your child with home-cooked meals, you'll be giving one of the highest forms of love a parent can offer. A valuable book for parents is "How to Raise a Healthy Child in Spite of Your Doctor", by Robert Mendelsohn. For specific help with food, see "Nourishing Traditions" by Sally Fallon. To understand how to manage the education of your child, see "Magical Child" by Joseph C. Pearce, and "Natural Learning" by Jane Evans, and "How to Be an Adult" by David Richo (I can't recommend these books enough).

Several thousand food chemicals exist today, and every year more are developed to stimulate food characteristics such as smell, colour, sweetness, crispness, increased shelf-life, shape, texture, etc.[149] As of 2004, the FDA listed 2,800 food additives and 3000 chemicals considered "safe" for consumption.

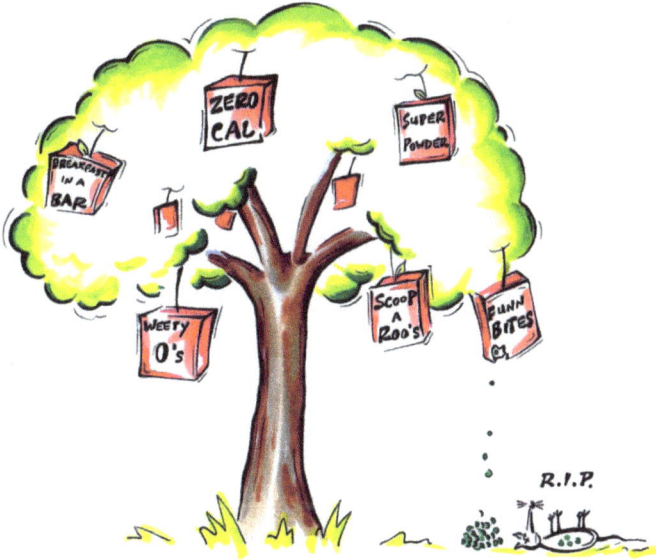

The sheer magnitude of chemicals and additives added to different foods makes it practically impossible to test for harmful synergistic effects. Many people have learned from chemistry class how baking soda and vinegar are inert when separate, but together they create a bubbling, fizzy mess – you can make a small volcano erupt by combining them! So, what happens when the "safe" chemical aspartame (which is not safe to begin with), from one food product, mixes with the "safe" yellow dye#5 of another, and "safe" potassium benzoate from another? No one knows. What happens to a person's health, happiness and vitality when mixtures of chemicals like these are consumed for years? No one knows!

Dr. Samuel Epstein is one of the most knowledgeable people in the world on correlations between chemicals and cancer. In his book, "The Politics of Cancer, Revisited", he states the following:

> *"Whenever it is announced that a chemical is carcinogenic in animals, there is usually an accompanying disclaimer that "the chemical has not been found to be harmful to humans". Every time you read this kind of statement in the press or hear it announced on the radio or television, you should mentally insert the word "yet".[150]*

"LABORATORY 101"   "HUMAN 101"

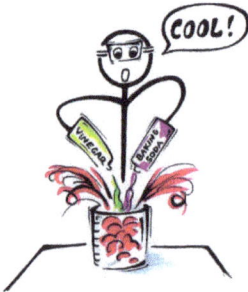
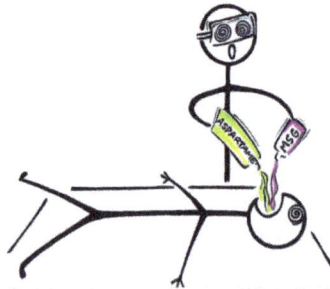

Initially, before a chemical is discovered to indeed cause damage to the health of animals, only short-term tests are carried out in search for any measurable disease caused. If the short term study does not find disease in the animal, the additive is deemed "safe" and added to the GRAS list: "Generally Regarded as Safe" to be eaten by humans.[151]

If you're a food manufacturer and want to increase the crispness of your product, you can just search through the GRAS list for "crispyness-making chemicals".

Government food agencies do not require GRAS list chemicals to be clearly labeled on the ingredient list of foods. Instead, chemicals are grouped together under the heading: "Natural Flavours", "Spices", or similar catch-all words.[152]

Thousands of additives have been deemed GRAS, yet the Environmental Working Group (which looks out for the public's health and well-being) provides several scientific studies that show detrimental health effects of many GRAS chemicals, ranging from inflammation to cancer.[153]

Food manufacturers can use as many GRAS additives as they wish, without having to label them individually. Thus, seeing the term "natural flavour" on an ingredient list means any number of additives may be in that product. Consider the "natural flavour" found in a typical strawberry milkshake:

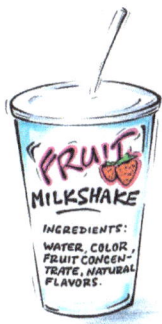

Natural Strawberry Flavour

Amyl acetate, amyl butyrate, amyl valerate, anethol, anisyl formate, benzyl acetate, benzyl isobutyrate, butyric acid, cinnamyl isobutyrate, cinnamyl valerate, cognac essential oil, diacetyl, dipropyl ketone, ethyl butyrate, ethyl cinnamate, ethyl heptanoate, ethyl lactate, ethyl methylphenylglycidate, ethyl nitrate, ethyl propionate, ethyl valerbate, heliotripin, hydroxyphrenyl-2butanone (10% solution in alcohol), a-ionone, asobutyl anthranilate, isobutyl butrate, lemon essential oil, maltol, 40methylacetophenone, methyl anthranilate, methyl benzoate, methyl cinnamate, methyl heptane carbonate, methyl naplhthyl ketone, methyl salicylate, mint essential oil, neroli essential oil, nerolin, neryl isobutyrate, orris butter, phenethyl alcohol, rose, rum ether, y-undecalactone, vanillin, and solvent.[154]

Let's look at another example I grabbed off the shelf at a local grocery store, we'll call "Lunch Supreme".

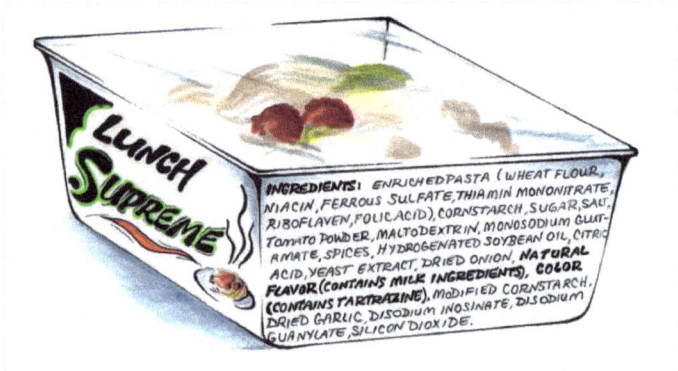

Counting the number of whole foods on the ingredient list in the picture above, we come up with two: garlic and onion. In addition to chemicals like MSG (monosodium glutamate), refined sugar and hydrogenated oil, Lunch Supreme has "Natural Flavour" and "Colour", which could mean any number of additives from the GRAS list.

As explained, some food additives are far worse than others. Aspartame for example, is an artificial sweetener that has "zero calories" and accounts for 85% of the health complaints filed to the FDA.[155] Despite these complaints, food manufacturers continue to add it to food products. Research has demonstrated that when aspartame is ingested, it causes neurons in the brain to fire repeatedly until they "burn out" and die.[156] Aspartame has been highly correlated with the development of brain cancer, and many children have died from seizures within weeks after beginning to drink diet pop.[157] After these horrific effects of aspartame were discovered, food manufacturers deceptively changed its name to Aminosweet.

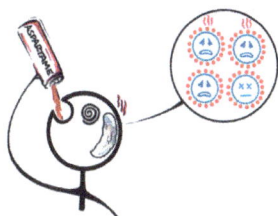

Monosodium Glutamate (MSG) is another common food additive that's highly stressful to our body. It is used to fatten laboratory rats to study potential weight loss drugs,[158] and is known to cause brain and liver damage.[159] It is found in many fast foods, and processed foods, and is commonly found right on the shelf of the local grocery store.

It is almost impossible for a chemical on the GRAS list to be removed if it is damaging the health of consumers. For example, if you have a headache and you're sure it came from a chemical within the ingredient list of a food product you ate, you'll need to prove it with your own self-funded research. Then you must write to the appropriate government agency, and submit your research study. Even then, only with multiple reports from other people presenting similar studies, may the food additive in question be removed.

How do we sort through this mess of chemicals and additives? Eat whole organic food and drink pure water (organic fruits and vegetables, free range meat, wild caught fish, organic oils and grass fed butter). You can experiment with small quantities of nuts and non-gluten-containing grains such as rice or corn, but watch for symptoms in your body, such as low energy, bloating, or unhealthy stools. For more guidance on food choices, see the book, "How, to Eat, Move, and Be Healthy!", by Paul Chek.

TIP
Put a face behind your food source: Find a local private health-food grocery store, or find a farmer and meet them in person. Purchase all your food, if possible, from them – put your money into the hands of people who care about you, humanity, animals, and our ecosystems. It's an investment that will pay you back in the long run, which you can feel good about too.

▶ Suggested Videos
Labels Matter – Just label it! (www.justlabelit.org)
www.youtube.com/watch?v=qnntmIWl5Xw

Sweet Misery: A Poisoned World
www.youtube.com/watch?v=toKyRlpmG7A

The Dangers of MSG – "Your Brain's Biggest Enemy" Part 2A
www.youtube.com/watch?v=NWt7JgEzjrU

The Hidden Source of Belly Fat: MSG Monosodium Glutamate
www.youtube.com/watch?v=KkBWi3G9qM0

Gluten: What You Don't Know Might Be Killing You
www.youtube.com/watch?v=yLJSmJ0bMlk

Aspartame Name Change
www.youtube.com/watch?v=DTRTnSTjvPQ

CINDY'S CANCER REVERSAL

I was diagnosed with stage 4 lung cancer back in May of 2021. Throughout the whole journey of me getting diagnosed, I was filled with fear - constant fear: "You have to get the chemo.. You have to do this… It's aggressive."

I started out with traditional chemo, and then I was moved to targeted therapy, which was chemo drugs. In March of this past year, I was told that the targeted chemo wasn't working anymore either. They had one last drug they were going to try, which would affect my central nervous system. I was going to have all these terrible side effects, it probably wouldn't work for much longer than a year, and there really wasn't anything else left in the pipeline. This last message was grim, and I pretty much told my family that I would rather just come home and live out my time I had left, versus being affected cognitively, or be impacted with short term memory loss and things like that.

A friend of mine reached out to me and suggested I talk to Paul. I had one session with Paul and my fear instantly changed to hope, and completely turned me around. Two weeks after my session I went to the Mayo Clinic for my appointed scan to help determine my next treatment approach, but my lung tumour was completely gone.

From the bottom of my heart, I'm so thankful and grateful for Paul.

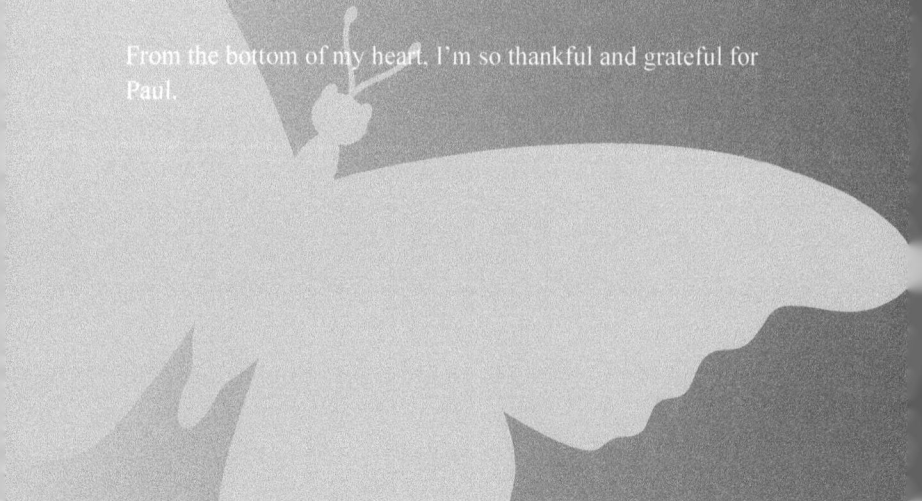

11

CHRONIC STRESS CAN TRIGGER CANCER

Modern-day living can be challenging at times – and often, chronically. Regardless of age, race or gender, some form of chronic stress affects almost everyone today: worries about money, unresolved relationship challenges, lack of meaning in life, lack of freedom, judgment of self or others, etc. If these challenges are not transcended through positive change and personal growth, can the buildup of stress in our body lead to the development of cancer cells?

Only positive change resolves stress, but change can be difficult for multiple reasons. One reason is that it takes energy to change, and people often are already overwhelmed or exhausted prior to encountering a life-challenge that demands their energy.

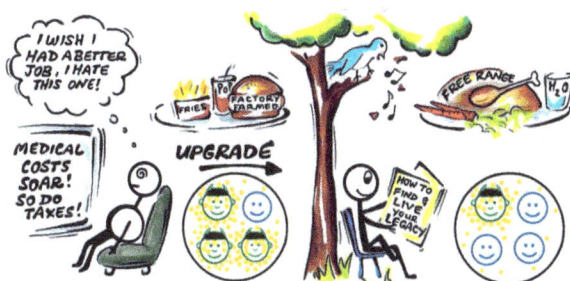

Another reason change can be difficult is because it requires a reconstruction of our "self". Said another way, who we are has likely been substantially influenced and shaped by society or other factors that don't align with our highest-potential. The society which shaped who we "are", is not healthy (recall that when a child is born today they enter a race of humans who have a 50% chance of developing cancer). Cancer and other forms of compromised health have become a "normal part of life" in society. Thus we must consciously redesign our "self" and life so that we live by values which create health and well-being – not chronic unfulfilled needs and stress.

NOTE: As you heal, you may no longer resonate with many of the norms and values of society, or certain people (this is an often challenging but normal part of healing).

To live fully, experiencing happiness and health, with meaning in our lives, we must understand that we all have human needs – and fulfilling our needs must be our priority. Health is the natural result of the fulfilment of our needs. Cancer is the natural result of important needs not being fulfilled, chronically. Some of our needs are:

- Sleep and rest
- Play
- Freedom
- Having purpose in life
- Eating real organic food
- Drinking water
- Moving our body
- Doing what makes us happy and knowing what that is.
- Loving ourselves – accepting, acknowledging, and feeling self-worth
- Connection with others who resonate with us, and share similar values
- Harmonious relationships, or relationships which are growing
- Expressing our Real Self, in accordance with our honest desires, emotions, and fears
- Living in a nourishing, peaceful (at least mostly!) environment
- Fresh, unpolluted air
- And more

That may seem like a lot to accomplish, but what else is worth striving for in this life other wholeness and a life worth living for? Until we create a life that fulfills our needs adequately, we cannot stay healthy long-term, or heal. **It's not necessary to accomplish everything right away – just moving in the direction of accomplishing our goals is healing.** Until we focus on what matters (our needs), we will likely live life through a disease-creating template often acquired by society or childhood, that wasn't even consciously agreed to by us; a template that can and does, in many cases, lead to cancer.

If we aren't investing our time and energy into the fulfilment of our needs, and the accomplishment of our dreams, it often means we are instead fulfilling someone else's needs, and energizing someone else's dream, and that dream may not even be life-affirmative for ourselves and others.

Society may have taught us to eat in a way that destroys our body over time. Or, we may have been taught that the only way to get what we need in life, or feel self-worth from, is by sacrificing ourselves in some way, or controlling others. We may have been taught to strive mainly for money and set our real passions aside because of a belief that our passions "won't make us successful". We may have been instilled with a belief system that leads us to being afraid of ever taking risks, living freely, and becoming independent.

TIP

To prevent or reverse cancer, it is essential to become clear about what makes you happy, and take actions to fulfill that happiness. What makes you happy? When do you genuinely feel happiness? Maybe you need more rest so that you have enough energy to be happy with what's within your grasp already? Maybe you need to try new things to discover what

For many, the healing or change process may at first feel overwhelming. It's a process that just needs to start – that is all. No rush, just keep at it. Significant changes can be scary – it's like a mini-death of our ego. However, if we dare to face our fears and begin the process of change, life can become more beautiful than imagined, and we can heal. From my extensive experience working with cancer clients, I am 100% certain that **the high incidence of cancer is the result of individuals being "stuck" in unresolved sources of chronic stress, that they have a hard time breaking free of.**

According to Edward Lytton, 19th century politician, poet, playwright, and novelist:

> *"We live longer than our forefathers, but we suffer more from a thousand artificial anxieties and cares. They fatigued only the muscles, we exhaust the finer strength of the nerves."*[160]

In the past, stress certainly existed, but the amount of chronic stress (especially psychological and emotional stress) has increased significantly with the dawn of the technological era. Many Indigenous societies, for example, experienced low levels of psychological stress because they lived in harmony with nature, they were more capable of fulfilling their needs compared to humanity today, and they experienced a lot of freedom (for example, children grew up naturally – a school system did not exist).

1800

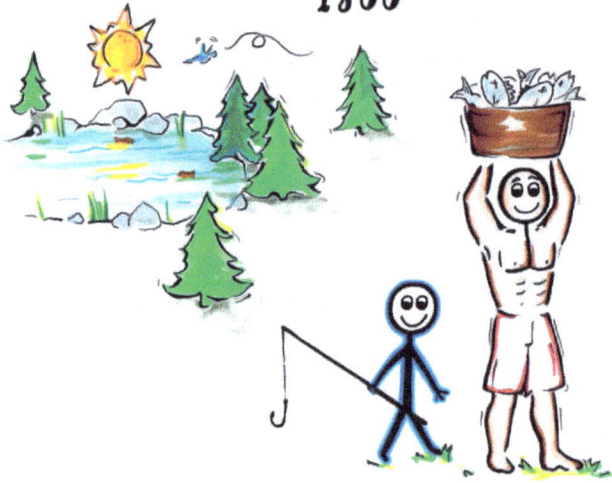

2012

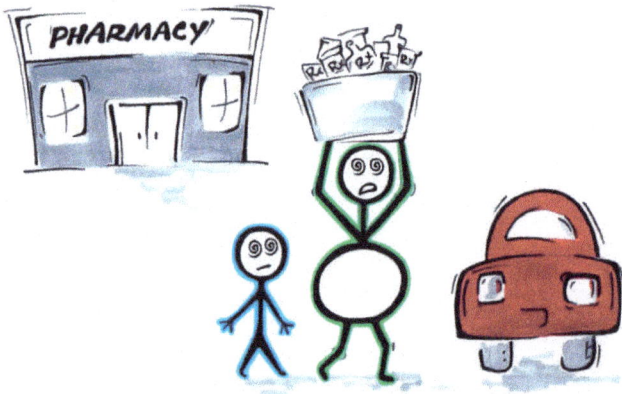

Today, many individuals in developed nations have only rare or minor experiences of connection to nature, because society influences us from a young age to spend most of our time indoors being "productive"(children are put into school at a young age, and for the first 15 – 20 years of their life, for the most part, they learn to first prioritize accomplishments, money and social status, not happiness, connection to nature, foundational health principles, freedom, self-love, discovering who they are, and living with purpose).

Whereas humans of the past found value in the natural world – not the material one. Their quality of life was not linked to convenience or accumulation of "things"[161] – it was more about **the quality of connection to oneself, others and nature.** Stress was acute, not chronic, and freedom was high. An excellent book on Aboriginal customs is, "Voices of the First Day", by Robert Lawlor.

In "Ten Thousand Years from Eden", Charles Heizer Wharton, PhD, makes the following comment:

> *"For many of us, our major communication with nature is a trip to the local supermarket, mowing the grass or maybe a fall drive to look at the leaves. Our enormous medical expenses attest that society at large has lost its once healthy relationships with life-giving soil and traditional ways."[162]*

In the 1920s, a dentist named Weston A. Price carried out one of the most extensive studies on the health of indigenous people. For over 10 years, Dr. Price and his wife traveled to remote locations around the world in search of remaining societies not yet influenced by the values of modern civilization.[163] His book, "Nutrition and Physical Degeneration", documents the health of those untouched tribes remaining on our planet. The location of these tribes ranged from tropical to northern arctic environments. Not only did Price find exceptional health among every tribe he studied, he could not find a single one that even had a word for "cancer" in their spoken language.[164]

A collection of writings and speeches, titled "The Wisdom of the Native Americans", include some of the following quotes from Native American Chiefs:

> "Look at me – I am poor and naked, but I am the chief of the nation. We do not want riches, but we do want to train our children right. Riches would do us no good. We could not take them with us to the other world. We do not want riches. We want peace and love."
> ~Red Cloud

> "Love is something you and I must have. We must have it because without it we become weak and faint. Without love our self-esteem weakens. Without it, our courage fails. Without love we can no longer look out confidently at the world. We turn inward and begin to feed upon our own personalities, and little by little we destroy ourselves. With it, we are creative. With it, we march tirelessly. With it, and with it alone, we are able to sacrifice for others."
> ~Chief Dan George

> "Let us put our minds together and see what kind of life we can make for our children!"
> ~Sitting Bull[165]

Most of humanity is so caught up in the "rat race of life", that they have little time to appreciate or protect the things of real value, including themselves. Nature is being destroyed at an alarming rate.[166] More species are going extinct than ever before in history – approximately ten thousand per year.[167]

NOTE: From my observations, the grand majority of people do not know who or what they are supporting with their dollars when they spend money. They may buy lumber to build a deck, but have no idea the wood came from the clear-cutting of some of the oldest most beautiful trees on the planet, such as in British Columbia. The companies that sell the wood just keep cutting and cutting – they don't tell the customers to stop consuming or label their product properly to inform customers what they are contributing to, and most governments aren't taking responsibility for overseeing and successfully enforcing truly sustainable or moral practices.

Or, for example, people buy non-organic grains from a mono-crop farm, not realizing that their purchase has supported the pollution of the Earth's soil, water and air, and additionally, has destroyed the habitat and taken the lives of a variety of animals.

It is so critical to be conscious of how you help shape our world with money; how you make your money, and then who you give it to. Entire ecosystems are disappearing (with all the variety of life they contain), all in the name of increased consumption, materialism and greed. An important book on this subject is, "The Future of Life", by Edward O. Wilson.

TIP

Make time daily to disconnect from all the to-do lists and even the people in your life, and find a comfortable spot alone (or go for a walk), and simply practice being present where you are. Breathe consciously, and be silent. Watch, listen, smell and feel. The deeper you can take yourself into this experience on a consistent basis, the more your energy levels and mood will rise, and your heart rate, blood pressure, stress hormones, and blood glucose levels will stabilize. Your chances of developing cancer will lower, and your ability to reverse cancer if you have it, will increase. Aim for at least 20 minutes every day, preferably before you start your day.

NOTE: if you find this suggestion uncomfortable or even impossible to actual carry out, it may be because the experience will connect you to unresolved emotional stress, or un-faced fears. Simply sitting in silence for long enough, may bring you to tears (crying) because it can cause an uprising of suppressed emotional pain, or confront us with something we do not want to "look at". This is a good thing, because to resolve stress, it needs to be processed consciously and appropriate changes need to be made, and this very process is part of healing (discussed in great detail in Book 2).

For the last two million years, humans have spent 99% of their time as hunter-gatherers.[168] Hunting and gathering societies had developed a lifestyle that fulfilled their needs for nutrient-dense food without much time and effort, and they still had an enviable amount of leisure time leftover.[169] **Traditional Aboriginals are reported to have worked a few hours each morning hunting and gathering, and then spent the rest of the day playing games and relaxing with family and friends.[170]** Anthropologist Richard Lee, estimates that a Kung woman from the Kung Bushman of Africa, could gather enough food in one six-hour day to feed her entire family for three days.[171]

Developed nations whose rate of cancer is 150% higher than underdeveloped nations,[172] have obviously created a way of living that increases the chances of triggering cancer-growth. Simultaneously, the possibility of self-healing (reversing cancer through positive change of lifestyle and resolution of life-challenges) is still often not practiced, or taken seriously.

TIP

Deep-breathing meditation, (eg. - a practice of letting go of stress by consciously breathing through the nose, putting ourselves into a state of silent relaxation), can immediately improve homeostasis by lowering blood pressure, blood acidity, and blood glucose.[173 174 175] Contrast a state of meditation with the detrimental physiological effects of traffic jams, or feeling pressure to pay off credit card debt, or feeling trapped in a job, relationship or life-challenge that drains our energy and takes away happiness. Meditation alone cannot solve these problems, but it can help support us through the process of change. Meditation is a valuable tool to de-stress, and through the self-connection it allows, can provide us with insights on what we need to take action on to make our life more whole.

Chronic stress that can result from relationship challenges is one of the most common causes of cancer that I see in my practice, working with cancer patients. Most people have learned skills to earn a paycheck, but not skills for building and growing healthy relationships. School does not teach how to have a healthy relationship or other important life skills, yet often replaces parents as the main source of child rearing. This kind of upbringing is likely a major contributing factor to 45% of marriages ending in divorce,[176] while many of the "successful" marriages are not necessarily devoid of unresolved challenges either. Relationships must continue to grow together to remain healthy and fulfilling. If not, partners can get emotionally "stuck" in stress, unfulfilled, disconnected from each other, and themselves. **Relationship challenges left unresolved, lead to one of two possibilities: the end of the relationship, or chronic stress and disease (which can include cancer).**

NOTE: Sometimes relationships are meant to end, which can be incredibly painful and hard to accept, but if growing together has not been possible, ending the relationship is the growth.

TIP

Sometimes all that's needed to maintain or restore harmony in relationships with others, is taking more time for yourself. After a long days work, spend at least 20 minutes alone in freedom. Once you establish a daily routine that provides you with a dose of self-time, you'll likely notice that you have more love to give to others, and you'll be able to manage stress better if it arises. You'll likely feel more inspired to share time with others, rather than feeling obliged to.

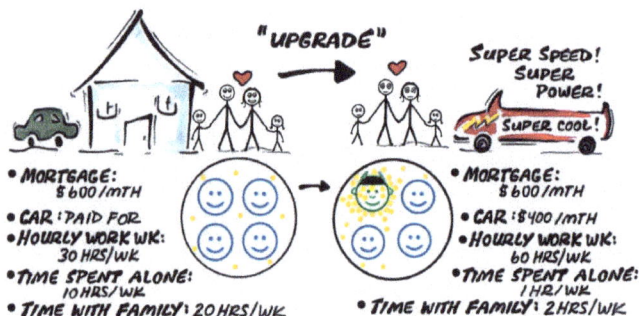

Here is a hypothetical example of a relationship challenge: One partner has had a long stressful day, and comes home hungry and grumpy, with low energy. As a result, they have "nothing to give" to their partner or others (such as patience or an ear to listen) because they're energetically drained and first need to fulfill their own needs. They may have an underlying feeling of irritation. In a state like that, it doesn't take much to instigate an argument. One or both partners can end up feeling resentment, regret, or any number of psychological stressors from the interaction.

Whether or not either partner realizes it, the consequential activated stress response floods each partners bloodstream with glucose. Additionally, there is now "tension in the air" due to an unresolved issue. Both partners may decide to "let it go", but unless the issue was truly resolved they are really just suppressing emotional pain. **Both partners will have suffered damage somewhere in their body, due to the physiological effects of psychological stress.**

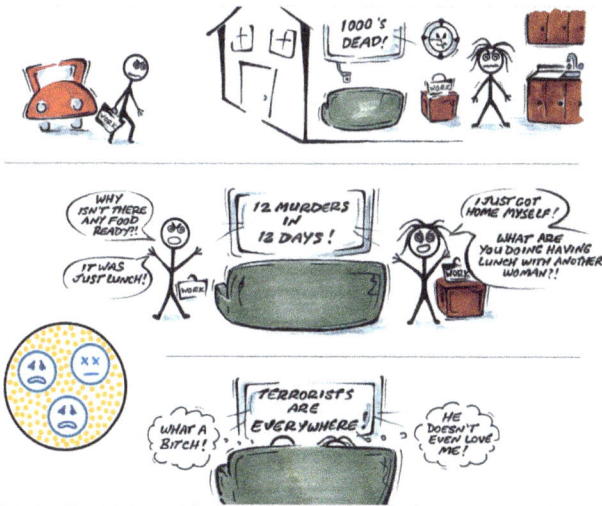

If you're unsure whether you have too much stress in your life, or whether you've become stuck in an unresolved challenge, look at the following list of common symptoms of chronic psychological stress:

• Weight gain
• Erectile dysfunction

- Heart disease and stroke
- Headaches and migraines
- Excessive fatigue
- Weakened immune system
- High blood pressure
- High cholesterol
- Muscle and joint pain
- Constipation
- Depression
- Insomnia
- Anxiety
- CANCER[177]

Only positive **change** heals. If you need help to improve your reality, or resolve a life-challenge, consider hiring one of my trained Root Cause Practitioner Coaches (www.rootcauseinstitute.com).

Indeed, psychological stress has a direct effect on our body. For example, to properly digest food and absorb nutrients, we must be relaxed and feel safe. A common side-effect of chronic psychological stress is irritation of the digestive tract, which can lead to loose stools or constipation.[178] Chronic stress over-stimulates the sympathetic branch of our nervouss system, and at the same time suppresses the calming digestion-supporting effect of the parasympathetic branch.

Since psycho-emotional stress has an impact on our physical body, it is extremely important to build healthy, loving relationships (by learning how to grow together through challenges). Healthy relationships are one of the most important aspects of life.

It will never be possible to avoid stress altogether, and no relationship is ever perfect, but it is still essential that a relationship grows (or ends if it can't grow) to avoid getting "stuck" in unresolved challenges. We can strive to constantly evolve ourselves alongside our partner – then, our human journey and relationships become more exciting, meaningful and fruitful, and our control over our health (and cancer) rises significantly.

ROOT CAUSE PRACTITIONER TRAINING

The Root Cause Practitioner Level One course has been, for lack of a more accurate way to describe it, life changing for me, both personally and professionally. The live, personal, and deeply insightful information, teachings, and experience-sharing that Paul so gracefully organized this course around, has been so deeply soul supporting for me in such an unparalleled way.

Within one to two months of completing the Level one course, I have been able to absorb, process and integrate the material in such a way that I have been able to guide myself significantly deeper into my own self healing process, using this unique, highly effective, life changing method of true healing.

The entire world truthfully needs to discover Paul and his work, as if they did, we would all have the available tools to understand how to go inwards, reach the inner depths of our true selves, acknowledge and release our unresolved traumas, and live soulfully and fully in the most healing way possible.

With sincere gratitude,
-*Jeremy*
Naturopathic Doctor

12

CANCER'S LOCATION IS NOT RANDOM

You may have heard the statement "everyone has cancer cells in their body at all times"; this statement points to the possibility that cancer is a natural process occurring in our body that can be activated or deactivated. However, the escalation of cancer cell development is obviously a serious problem, and very likely is directly related to factors and circumstances in our life.

Not only does cancer develop for a reason, it also appears in specific locations of the body for a reason. **Cancer grows where chronic stress has accumulated in the body, and where that stress accumulates is determined by factors in our daily reality.**

There are four main categories of stress that a human being can experience, which can summate together: physical, mental, emotional, and spiritual. For example, emotional pain from losing someone we love(grief) can cause physiological stress in our lungs, while physical harm from smoking cigarettes can add more stress to our lungs. These are two different sources of stress from different categories, yet both affect the same location of the body. If both of these sources of stress are present at the same time, their stress will summate (intensify) at the location of the lungs.

You can develop cancer in the lungs without ever having smoked a cigarette. A common cause of lung cancer that I have discovered in my practice over the years, is the suppression of emotional pain that has resulted from the loss of a loved one (unresolved grief).

From my continual observations and experiences with clients, here are some examples of potential root causes of cancer:

1. Physical: for example, liver cancer is correlated with chronic exposure to chemicals.[179] Our liver filters chemicals from our bloodstream and has a limit to what it can manage.

2. Mental: such as from chronic thought-patterns related to deep emotional wounding from the past; or perpetual fears of the future – which can cause cancer in the brain.

3. Emotional: such as anger or resentment from trying to control something that is out of our control; or allowing someone to repeatedly harm us emotionally, without setting a healthy boundary – this can lead to liver or ovarian cancer.

4. Spiritual. In truth, **I believe the deepest root cause of all cancer is spiritual:**

Let's consider the example of liver cancer from chronic exposure to chemicals. It may appear that chemicals are indeed the root cause, and this is true from one perspective. However, the deeper root cause is the subconscious, or conscious choice to stay in a job which causes the repeated exposure to chemicals. In this example, to reverse cancer one might need to detoxify their liver, however, their cancer would only come back – if they continued to be exposed to the same chemicals. The question then is, why are they staying in the job, despite the exposure? The answer might be, "because I have no choice". This is the spiritual component I am referring to – the belief that they have no choice. This belief, "having no choice" is often rooted in fear of the future. In this case, it may be fear that if they quit their job and search for a new one, such as working for a more ethical and environmentally-conscious business that does not produce such toxic chemicals, they may not get a job or they may not make enough money. **Fear is powerful, and it can keep a person stuck in a harmful situation, while simultaneously preventing them from choosing and pursuing a life that would be good for them.**

Hence, the spiritual challenges of life are the greatest and most difficult to face because they always involve difficult decisions, fear, and life-changing events.

Spiritually speaking, **creating a life we want, is a moment-to-moment act of creation itself.** In other words, we can only achieve the goals we choose, and pursue. The deepest root cause of cancer in the example above, is not the chemicals – but rather the **fear and beliefs that leads to the choice NOT to remove ourselves from the chemicals and job that is harming us.**

Cancer Develops in Specific Organs

There is a reason why cancer develops more in certain parts of the body than others. For example, breast and lung cancer are the most common forms of cancer, and next is cancer of the colon.[180] What these statistics really represent, is that stress factors which effect the breast tissue or the lungs, are two of the most common stress-factors in our society today. Next, are stress-factors that affect the colon, and so on, with all other cancers.

Physically speaking, different chemicals damage different

parts of the body, contributing to cancer.[181] In the list below, a strong correlation to cancer is shared amongst the following groups of people:

- Cancer of the nose is highest among woodworkers (likely due to the commonly shared exposure to wood glues).
- Cancer of the larynx is highest among machine tool operators.
- Cancer of the salivary glands is highest among the armed forces.
- Cancer of the liver is highest among plastic workers.
- Cancer of the pancreas is highest among coal miners.
- Cancer of the brain is commonly associated with the consumption of Aspartame or Aminosweet, found it diet pop and other processed-foods.[182]
- Commercial farmers who grow crops with pesticides and other chemicals have the highest rates of cancer of the following: Hodgkin's disease, leukaemia, non-Hodgkin's lymphoma, multiple myeloma, and cancers of the lip, stomach, prostate, skin (nonmelanotic), brain, and connective tissues.[183 184]

The reason cancer occurs in specific parts of the body has to do with how our nervous system responds to stress.

Blood flow regulation, and bioelectric functions (eg. electrical impulses in the brain, heart and muscles) are key aspects which our nervous system regulates.[185] The two branches of our nervous system (sympathetic and parasympathetic) manage our physiology by prioritizing different needs in different parts of the body, at different times. For example, if pain or damage occurs in our body, the sympathetic nervous system (SNS) responds by expanding specific blood vessels, increasing blood flow to those areas, to deliver more oxygen, nutrients, immune cells and energy (glucose) which are needed for the repair process of the body.[186] Simultaneously, our parasympathetic branch (PNS) does the opposite – restricting blood flow to less important areas of the body (at that time).

Increased blood flow to a particular area of the body causes swelling and redness (inflammation). Chronically inflamed areas of the body are associated with the development of cancer cells. [187]

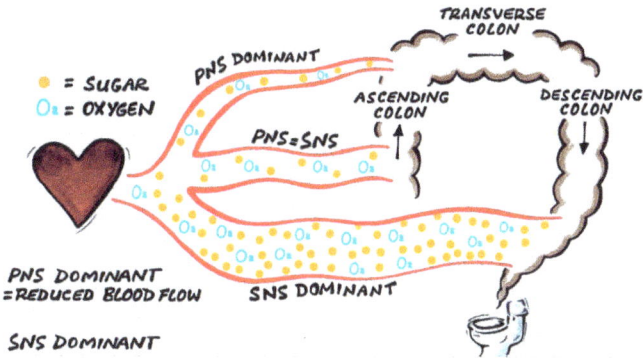

Here are some examples demonstrating the association between inflammation and cancer:

Example 1: Lung Cancer

When we breath polluted air, our body's initial response may be a cough or sneeze to expel the chemicals. However, if that response fails to solve the problem (because we don't stop the pollution or escape from it), a wound will begin to form in the lungs. Our body knows how to heal, but that wound can never fully heal if the source of the problem is not resolved. Our body is thus forced to launch a continuous inflammatory response in an attempt to repair the wound. Recall that this response increases blood flow to the lungs, carrying immune cells, oxygen, glucose and nutrients to the damaged area, to support detoxification and repair.[188] If the exposure to pollution continues, inflammation in the lungs will also continue, along with the associated side effects such as damage to cells caused by the dehydrating effects of excess glucose.

While pollution is causing chronic inflammation (and therefore increased blood flow) in a person's lungs, other sources of stress may also be present in their life. These secondary sources of stress may be psychological (fear, despair, grief, etc), which also activate the stress response, causing blood glucose surges. These secondary factors lead to further glucose damage in the already chronically inflamed lung tissue.

Another factor that makes the chronically inflamed areas susceptible to glucose damage is the degree to which our diet causes glucose surges (discussed in earlier chapters). Each meal consumed that triggers a blood glucose surge, will result in glucose damage at an already inflamed area of the body.

The longer any wound takes to heal, the more exposure it has to potential glucose damage. The availability of nutrients in our body required to repair the wounded area is one factor that determines the speed at which our body can heal any wound. **Thus, a diet high in nutrients will aid the wound-healing process.**

Consider the following possibility: while our body attempts to heal the wounded lung tissue, it can only cope for a certain amount of time before cancer cells are triggered to grow, the result of a last-resort survival mechanism. If enough dehydration damage from excess glucose occurs in the lungs, our body will begin growing cancer cells which will absorb the excess glucose. This may provide us more time to solve the root cause of the problem (pollution, unresolved grief, or both).

If the root cause of the inflammation is not addressed, the body will be pushed further into a state of survival, developing more cancer cells, as it attempts to manage the perpetual damage at the inflamed location. If we eliminate the cause(s) (pollution, psychological stress – especially grief, as mentioned, which is associated with the lungs), and any dietary factors causing glucose surges, our body can finally repair the area. At a certain point in the successful repair and regeneration process, cancer cells will no longer be of purpose in the body and can be deactivated. As healing completes, inflammation will cease, and cancer cells will disappear.

Example 2: Colon Cancer

In Chapter 8, we discussed how gluten found in most grains can damage the intestinal tract due to chronic inflammation, which it often causes. While the colon is inflamed, it is now more susceptible to the damaging dehydrating effects of excess blood glucose. As with the lungs, if any other secondary sources of stress occur simultaneously which also affect the colon, damage at the colon will summate. Examples of psychological stress that affect the colon, which I continue to observe in my practice, are stress about money, family, or social circles. If the problem persists, the body may be forced to produce cancer cells in the colon which absorb and thereby reduce the damage from excess blood glucose.

To reverse cancer in the colon, the individual must address physical and psycho-emotions sournces of stress such as: eliminate gluten from one's diet and avoid other foods and drinks which cause significant blood-glucose surges or inflammation in the diegestive tract; and resolve any stressful psychological factors that are causing glucose surges, such as those mentioned above.

NOTE: when trying to uncover the source of stress related to the onset of cancer, it's important to also look into the past, which may contain experiences that have led to unresolved emotional stress today, prior to the diagnosis (recall that cancer can be growing in the body months or even years before an official diagnosis). When all of these factors are resolved, the body can then have a chance to successfully complete the repair and regeneration process and deactivate both the inflammatory response and cancer cell production. Cancer cells can then be broken down and eliminated by the body.

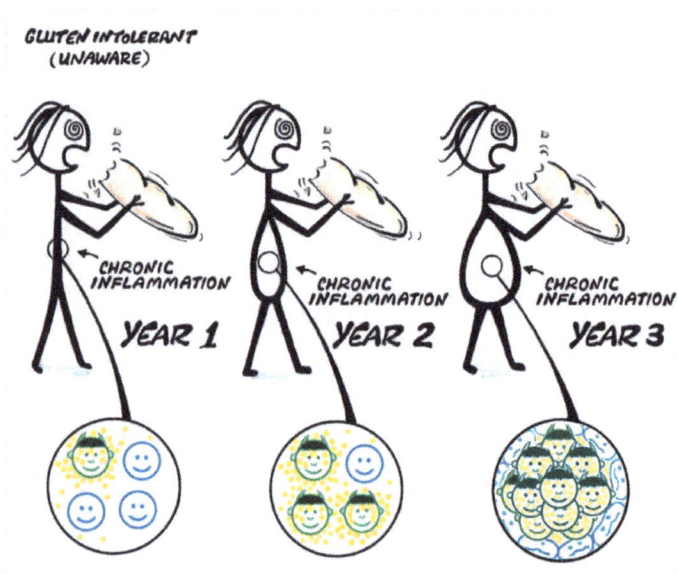

GLUTEN INTOLERANT (UNAWARE)

CHRONIC INFLAMMATION — YEAR 1

CHRONIC INFLAMMATION — YEAR 2

CHRONIC INFLAMMATION — YEAR 3

Infections

Research shows that chronic infections are strongly correlated with the development of cancer in specific locations of the body.[189] For example, the bacterial infection, H. Pylori, is associated with stomach cancer; Hepatitis C infection, with liver cancer,[190] and Human Papillomaviruses with cancer in the sex organs.[191] To reverse cancer in these examples, one needs to eradicate the infection by addressing what's causing the infection, and also resolve blood glucose factors. (NOTE: an area of the body will only develop an infection if it has already been compromised due to stress of some kind).

Not every stress nor every bout of inflammation will cause cancer. For example, if you step on a nail, it will cause stress and inflammation in your foot. While inflamed, your foot will be vulnerable to blood glucose damage, but because the event is not repetitive, your body can usually complete the healing process within days or weeks, and the inflammation and wound will mend and disappear.

Carrying Emotional Stress

Fear affects our physiology in significant (and detrimental) ways.[192] Fear is so powerful that it can cause us to lose consciousness, such as when a person who is afraid of needles, passes out when they decide to get one. Consider the fear of public speaking some people may experience as a tightening sensation in their stomach. In these two examples, fear is experienced until it's faced and dissolved; either the person is exempt from the needle, or gets the needle, and then the event is over. In the case of public speaking, once an individual faces their fear (speaks in front of an audience), over time their fear can transform into confidence. Until a fear is resolved, it continues to cause physiological stress, and can keep us "stuck" in life, preventing us from making choices that lead to fulfilment of our needs.

Fear and stressful emotions trigger the stress response, and can eventually lead to the development of cancer cells when experienced chronically. IMPORTANT NOTE: Suppression of emotions by "thinking positively", or "trying to forget about it", is not a solution – the body still carries the stress but now it becomes harder to resolve because you are less conscious of it.

In her book, "The Subtle Body", Cyndi Dale shares the following:

> *"Traditional Chinese practitioners understand that emotions affect physiology... Each emotion influences a specific organ. Under normal conditions, this relationship helps someone respond to life-events, but when the emotions are excessive or underdeveloped, the body will eventually become sick. Excessive anger, for example, is dangerous to the liver and other parts of the body."[193]*

Here are some examples of common stressful emotions, that can damage our body, according to Karol K. Truman in "Feelings Buried Alive Never Die":[194]

1. Anger
2. Hate
3. Guilt
4. Resentment
5. Rejection/Abandonment
6. Need for Approval
7. Overwhelmed Burden

Cancer Develops in Specific Parts of our Organs

In addition to cancer occurring in specific locations of the body, cancer also begins growing in specific parts of organs (namely, **the sheath**). The outer layer of all organs and glands throughout our body is enveloped with a sheath of tissue which acts as a sieve – blood must first filter through it before it can reach the organ. Interestingly, ninety percent of all types of cancer begin growing within the sheath of our organs.[195] Perhaps this positions cancer cells to filter excess glucose from the blood before it reaches our organs.

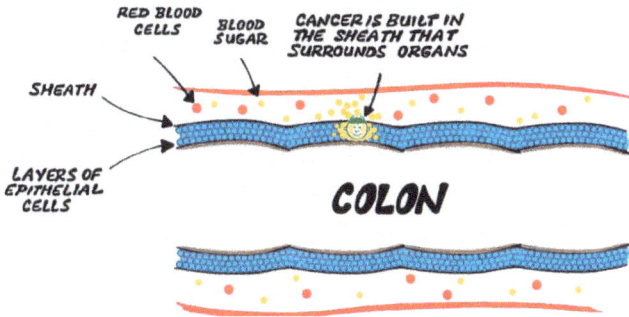

Cancer cells appear to grow in the body in specific locations and parts of organs for a reason: to reduce damage from excess blood glucose, granting us more time to solve whatever stress is chronically damaging us.

The location where cancer appears in the body provides important information that can be used to help identify the root cause, so that it can be resolved, allowing the growth of cancer cells to cease, and for cancer to eventually disappear.

SHEILA'S CANCER REVERSAL

I was diagnosed with Stage 3 endometrial cancer, which blew my mind because I always thought I was very healthy. However, I knew that if I came down with cancer, there was something not right and I needed to make a change.

I worked with Paul for 2 weeks, and when I started I was depleted – I had nothing. No energy. No motivation… And I could feel as we talked, and we peeled back the layers, more energy. With Paul's help I dealt with the things I needed to deal with and I learned the changes I needed to make. It was a gradual learning change – and with that came the energy, appreciation, and healing, healing, tremendous healing!

I am happy and life is no longer controlling me. And, I am cancer free.

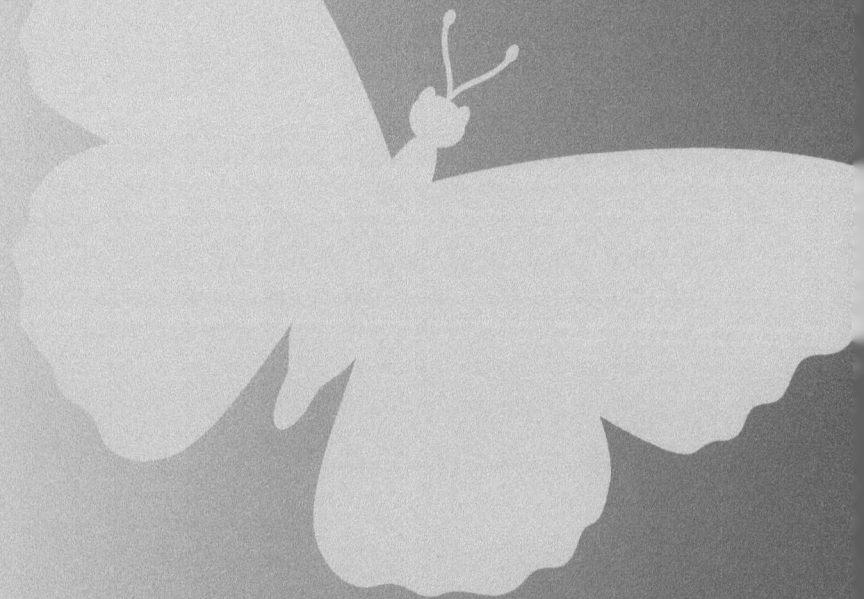

13

IT'S NOT OUR BODY'S FAULT

Our body begins as a single cell, and replicates trillions of times, building tissues, organs, bones, and more, forming an entire human body. Then, cells are repaired or replaced when needed. Every day, trillions of physiological processes and cellular operations take place within our body. For example, bone marrow alone, manufactures millions of red blood cells every second.[196]

The human body is an incredible system comprised of many systems – the immune, cardiovascular, reproductive, detoxification system, and many more – it is a miraculous creation. Even our skin is far more than a simple boundary-material; it creates vitamins from sunlight,[197] develops a tan to protect us from excess sun exposure, and sweats to cool us down. Our skin, and all systems of our complex body, somehow accomplish all of this and far more, while our body is constantly rebuilding anew, dozens of times throughout our life. We don't have to think to make any of this happen – its automatically taken care of by our body.[198]

If the human body is so extraordinary that it can accomplish all these processes simultaneously, how does it manage to make a cellular mistake like "cancer", and then fail to identify that error, and then proceed to allow that cell, to make millions more of itself? Let's take a closer look at the theory that cancer supposedly is a cellular error...

Researchers concluded in "A New Hypothesis for the Cancer Mechanism", **that the mathematical chance of cancer being the result of cellular errors is so low, that in a population of 8 billion people,** not a single person would have cancer.[199] Their findings also strongly suggest that **cancer is part of a complex survival-mechanism in our body:**

> *"Our proposed hypothesis is that cancer is a natural wound-healing-related process... if the cause of the wound or if the wound persists... the continuous wound healing process will lead to a clinical cancer mass. There is no system in nature to stop or reverse the wound healing process in the middle stage when the wound exists. The outcome of the cancer mechanism is either healing the wound or exhausting the whole system (death)."[200]*

As we discussed in the previous chapter, cancer develops in particular regions and parts of the body – parts that have been damaged or "wounded" by physical or psychological factors. If the body initiates cancer as part of a complex wound-healing process, it will continue indefinitely, until the source of the wound is resolved (the root cause of the cancer) or the body succumbs to the wound (death). In other words, **cancer will not naturally disappear unless we are able to resolve the factors that are perpetually wounding us physically and psychologically.**

There are infinite potential errors that could develop in one of the cells of our body. For example, deformed cell walls, misshaped DNA strands, incomplete receptor sites, broken enzymes, missing components, excess lipids; imbalances of any kind – the list is endless. Yet, the current mainstream theory of cancer essentially says that the body's of 1 in 2 people today, are accidentally making cancer cells; fully functioning cells with particular qualities, replicating on their own, absorbing large amounts of glucose from the bloodstream, and undetectable by our immune system?

The theory that cancer is a cellular mistake means our body must first fail to make a healthy cell, and then also fail to recognize the unhealthy cell was made – failing twice. This "failing" of our body is highly implausible. Our body has an intricate process for catching and correcting any cellular mistake: Our immune system "proofreads" each of our cells to identify potential imperfections. Next, it undergoes a second process called "mismatch repair", to catch any errors that may have been overlooked during proofreading. If an error is identified, that cell is repaired or destroyed (called apoptosis). According to the textbook, Cell and Molecular Biology, by Gerald Kelp:

> *"The job of proofreading is one of the most remarkable of all enzymatic activities and illustrates the sophistication to which our body's biological molecular machinery has evolved... Together, proofreading and mismatch repair reduce the overall observed error rate to about 0.000000001%.[201]*
> *In other words, there's a one-in-a-billion chance that our body will make any kind of cellular replication mistake, let alone a specific mistake that creates a complex, functioning cancer cell.* **We have a far greater chance of being struck by lightning, winning the lottery,[203] or being in a plane crash,[204] than our body forming cancer accidentally."**

The following two Figures show the manufacturing of cells in our body, which involves specialized immune cells that check for mistakes (proofreading and mismatch repair). If a cell with an error is found, that cell is destroyed through apoptosis. If a cell makes it through both checkpoints, it then takes its place as a healthy cell in our body:

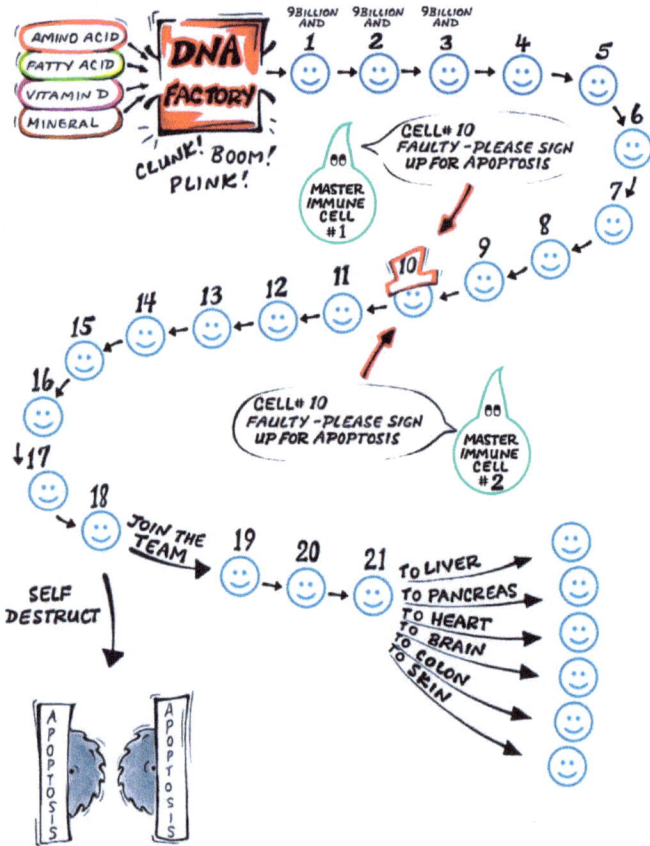

In the Figure above, both checkpoints find an error in Cell#10 (wearing the hat), and direct it to self-destruct (apoptosis) because the cell with a "hat" is noticed as an error.

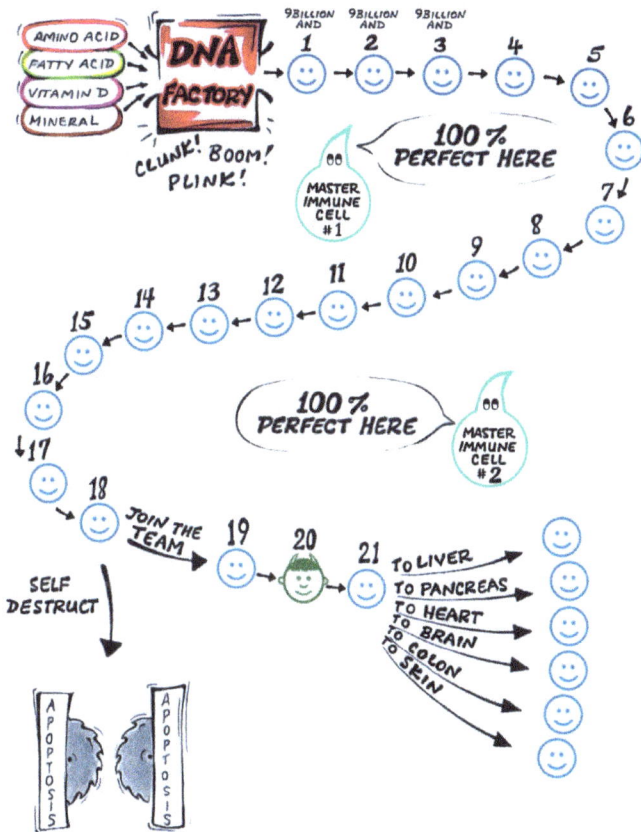

In this Figure, both checkpoints scan a cancer cell, yet do NOT tell the cell to self-destruct, and the cancer cell joins the body.

To understand how cancer develops, first we must understand how **enzymes work, because enzymes play a major role in both the establishment and function of cancer cells.**

How Enzymes Work

For a cellular change to take place in our body, an enzyme must combine with a substrate, which causes a reaction. Here is an analogy: Imagine walking up to the front door of your home; you unlock the door by inserting your key (enzyme) into the lock (substrate), which allows you to enter the house (re-action).

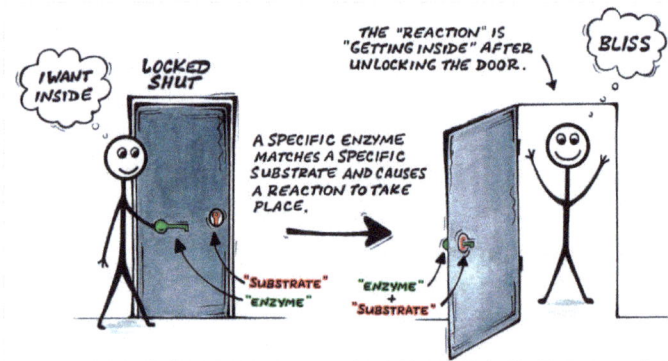

The real enzymatic reaction that takes place in our body is similar, but more impressive – the enzyme and substrate are energetically attracted to each other. So, as you approach your front door, your key is energetically pulled out of your pocket and flies to land and fit perfectly into the lock, and the door opens – that's how it works in our body.

The textbook, "Cell and Molecular Biology", describes the specificity of enzyme-substrate relationships:

> "That part of the enzyme molecule that is directly involved in binding the substrate is termed the "active site". The active site and the substrate have complementary shapes, enabling them to bind together with a high degree of precision, like the pieces of a jigsaw puzzle."[205]

In the textbook, "Human Physiology", author Dee Silverthorn describes the following important fact about enzymes:

> "*Without enzymes, reactions would depend on a random collision of molecules to bring them into alignment.*"[206]

In other words, the enzymatic relationships that cancer cells have with our normal cells are not random cellular mistakes. What are the chances of you unlocking the door of a neighbor's house with the key to your house? Pretty slim. **Cancer cells have several lock-and-key (perfect-fit) enzymatic relationships with our normal cells, and without these relationships, cancer cells could not exist.**

Cancer's Enzymatic Relationships With Our Body

Recall that insulin is a hormone that regulates glucose. Insulin and insulin receptors also form an enzyme-substrate relationship. When our blood contains too much glucose, our pancreas secretes the hormone insulin into our bloodstream; insulin molecules merge with the insulin receptors on the surface of cells throughout our body, causing an enzymatic reaction to take place that opens the door of the cells to allow glucose to enter. Recall that cancer cells have up to 23 times more insulin receptors compared to normal cells, which makes them capable of absorbing far more glucose.

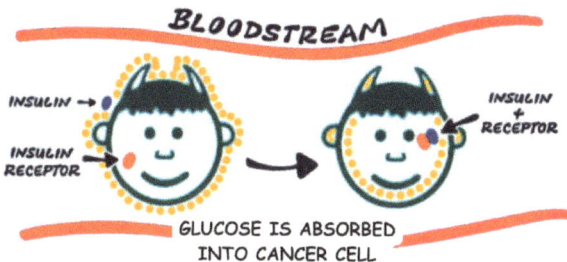

BLOODSTREAM

INSULIN →

INSULIN RECEPTOR

INSULIN + RECEPTOR

GLUCOSE IS ABSORBED INTO CANCER CELL

Our body is not an error-factory. More and more evidence suggests that cancer develops for deeper reasons than a "cellular error".

THE POWER OF THE 15 STEP PROCESS
(Taught in Root Cause Practitioner Level 1)

Dear Paul,

Since undertaking our 1:1 session, my life has changed.

I spent three days working through your 15 point emotional healing process, and recorded all of my self dialogue. Within 24 hours of our session my left (cancer) lung was starting to open up and I could feel air flowing in again.

I have also received your book and devoured it – I am keen to read book 2 when it's done.

Many thanks for your wisdom, healing and wonderful words.
With love and gratitude,
-Steve

14

OUR BODY FACILITATES THE GROWTH OF CANCER CELLS

In his book, "The Trophoblast and the Origins of Cancer", Oncologist Dr. Nicholas Gonzalez and colleagues share ground-breaking research on the natural, orchestrated events of our body's cancer cell development.

Dr. Gonzalez states "A cancer, to flourish, cannot make it on its own; it needs help, which it too often gets".[207] He is referring to the help that our normal cells give to cancer cells, which makes their development possible.

Enzymatic relationships exist for each of the steps required to embed a cancer cell in the sheath of an organ and also for its replication. The sheath has 3 layers: the epithelial layer, the basement membrane, and the stromal layer. A cancer cell takes up residence in the 3rd layer (stromal), after passing through the first two layers.

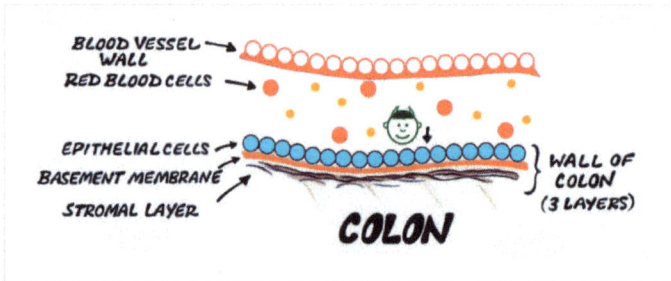

BLOOD VESSEL WALL
RED BLOOD CELLS

EPITHELIAL CELLS
BASEMENT MEMBRANE
STROMAL LAYER

WALL OF COLON (3 LAYERS)

COLON

Here is the step-wise process involved in the formation of a tumour:

Steps 1 & 2: Cancer cells have perfect-fit enzymatic relationships with both the 1st and 2nd layers of the sheath of our organs, which enable their entry into these layers.

Step 1

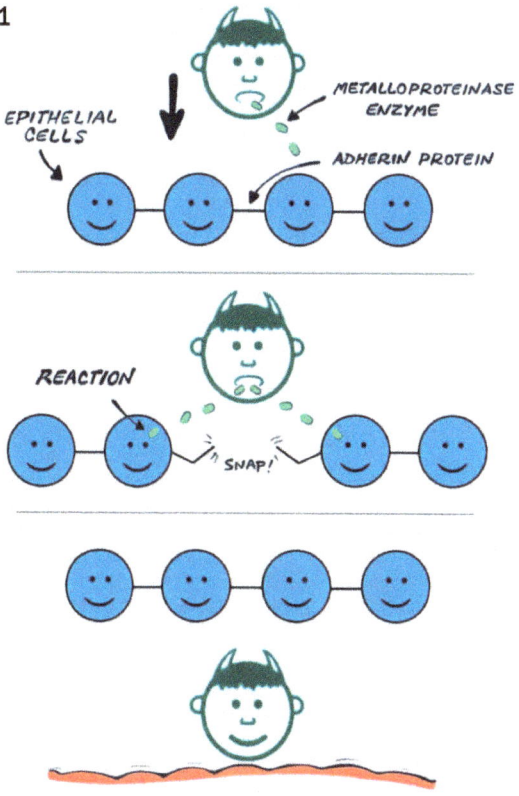

Step 1

The first layer of the sheath (the epithelial layer), is bound together by adherin proteins. Cancer cells release specific enzymes called metalloproteinases, which are a perfect match to the adherin protein receptor sites. This enzymatic reaction causes the bond to dissolve, creating an opening for the cancer cell to move through the epithelial layer.[208]

Step 2

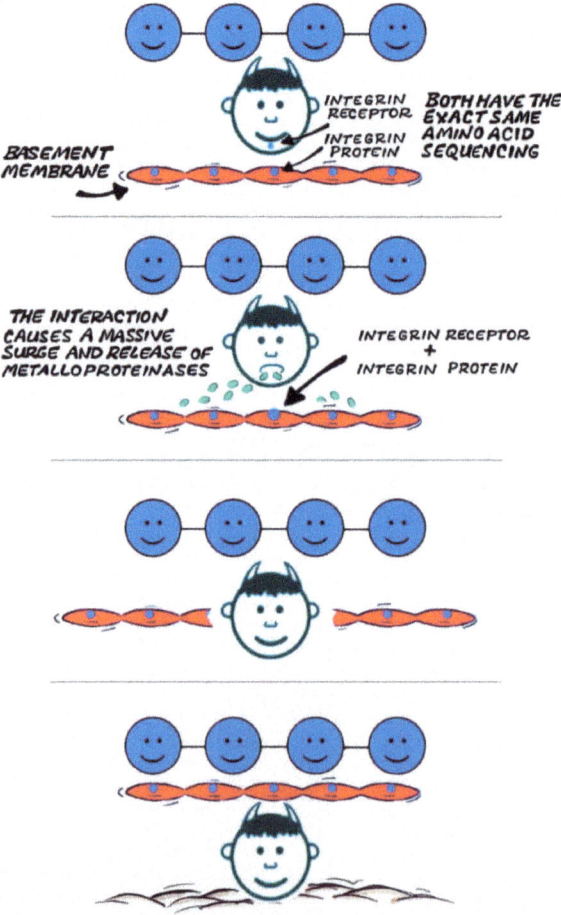

INTEGRIN RECEPTOR
INTEGRIN PROTEIN
BOTH HAVE THE EXACT SAME AMINO ACID SEQUENCING

BASEMENT MEMBRANE

THE INTERACTION CAUSES A MASSIVE SURGE AND RELEASE OF METALLOPROTEINASES

INTEGRIN RECEPTOR
+
INTEGRIN PROTEIN

Step 2

The middle layer of the sheath is called the basement membrane. Cancer cells are equipped with integrin receptors, which have the same amino acid sequencing as the basement membrane proteins. When the integrin receptors of the cancer cell merge with the basement membrane, it causes more metalloprotinase enzymes from inside the cancer cell to be released, creating openings in the basement membrane. The cancer cell now proceeds through the basement membrane.[209]

Step 3

The boundary line into the third layer of the sheath (the stromal layer), is dissolved by our body's own immune cells, allowing the cancer cell to pass through and embed into the last layer of the sheath.

Cancer cells do not have enzymes to dissolve the last layer (the stroma). Instead, at the stroma, an act of cooperation occurs between the cancer cell and our body's fibroblast and immune cells, which secrete their own enzymes to dissolve the stromal layer. This process allows the cancer cell to finish embedding fully into the sheath. Dr. Gonzalez states:

> *"Cancer cells cannot travel very far into the stroma without the direct cooperation of the extracellular matrix... Surprisingly, our own normal cells – including our normal immune cells – not only assist the invading cancer, but are necessary for the process to take place."[210]*

Step 4 & 5

Yet another unique relationship exists between cancer cells and immune cells, which protects both cancer and the sheath that it grows in.

Step 3

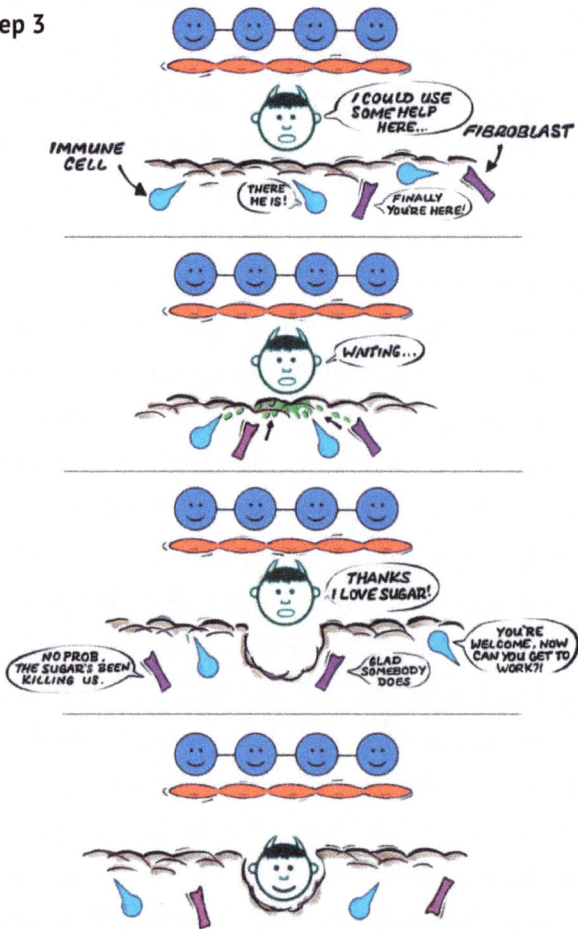

If the fibroblast cells of our immune system release too many enzymes when creating an opening for the cancer cell, the stromal layer could be severely damaged. Thus, cancer cells work cooperatively to release additional enzymes that regulate the quantity of the enzymes released by the immune and fibroblast cells. In the words of Dr. Gonzalez:

"With too much of the extracellular matrix [the sheath] destroyed, the tissue would fall apart along with the cancer cell... Cancer cells avoid such an outcome by releasing enzymes... so that the breakdown of the stroma and ECM proceeds sufficiently to allow migration, without total tissue annihilation. This coordination... must be very precise."[211]

Step 4&5

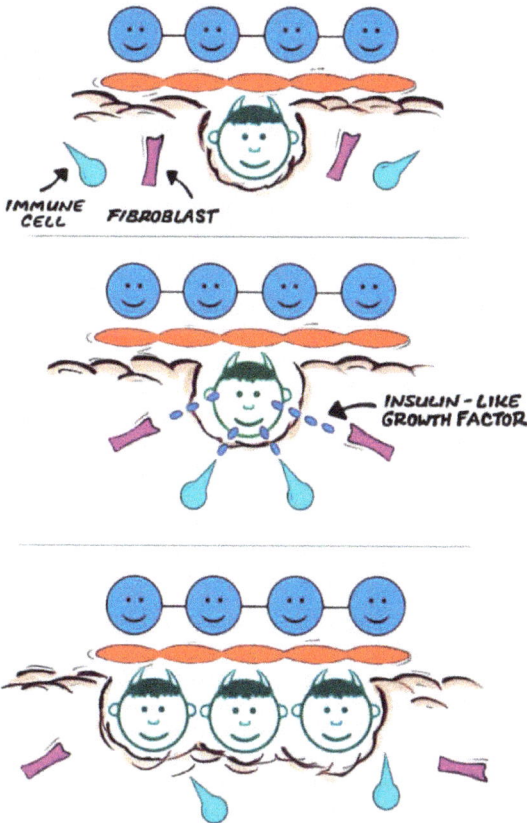

Once a cancer cell is embedded in the sheath, it multiplies. Again, our body's immune and fibroblast cells help – they stimulate the multiplication of the cancer cell by releasing their own growth hormone, IGF (Insulin-like Growth Factor). IGF causes the cancer cell to begin dividing.[212]

Cancer cells do NOT divide on their own – our immune system supports their growth!

Step 6

Next, our body builds a network of arteries to bring blood directly to the cancer cells. Epithelial cells from the first layer of the sheath, travel inwards until they reach the cancer cells. This creates pathways for blood flow. The following is a quote from the research of Murray and Lessey, in "Embryo Implantation and Tumour Metastasis: Common Pathways of Invasion and Angiogenesis":

"Cancer cells require a steady, substantial blood supply. Endothelial cells leave their home base, migrating through the sheath toward the tumour, creating small blood vessels along the way."[213]

The complex process of cancer cell development is clearly not an error. **Cancer cells will remain in our body, until the root cause is addressed, which is related to our lifestyle, and stressful life-challenges (occurring now or prior to diagnosis).**

Step 6

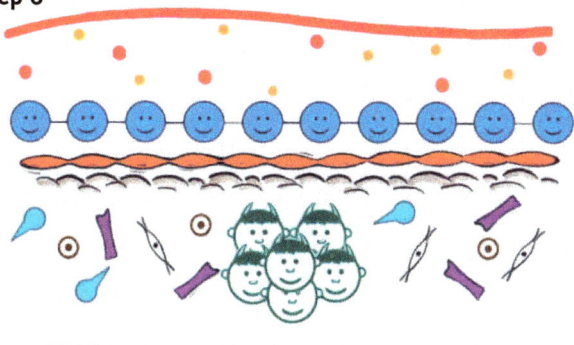

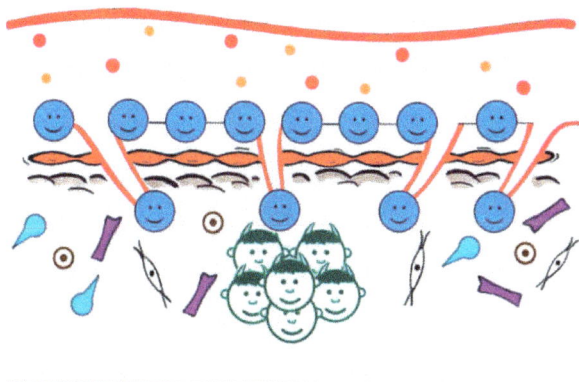

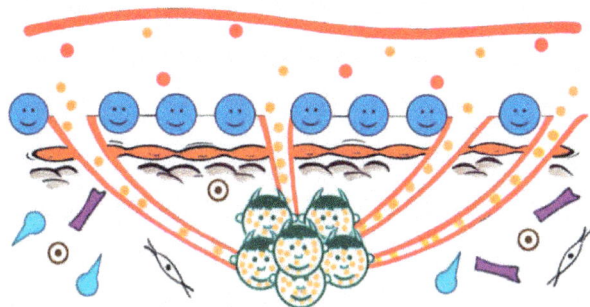

ELAINE'S CANCER REVERSAL

I have been plagued with skin cancer on my nose for over 20 years. I just had my third major surgery, and already in less than 6 weeks from surgery, it was obvious that the cancer had returned. When I realized my cancer has redeveloped faster than it ever had before, I reached out to Paul.

In a little over 2 1/2 weeks after my first appointment with Paul, the visible part of the cancer was totally healed.
If not for the scars from previous surgeries, no one would know I ever had skin cancer.

The daily routine of "processing" negative feelings from my childhood was exhausting. But I knew that if getting to the root causes of my chronic stress was necessary to heal my cancer and prevent further cancers in the future, I was determined to follow this journey. Imagine: Reversing Cancer. I had to experience it to believe it.

3 Months later:
Paul, I just wanted you to know that the skin cancer has not returned. Thank you so much for sharing your expertise. All is well!

15

YOU CAN PREVENT AND REVERSE CANCER

A cancer diagnosis is one of the scariest things you can experience in your lifetime. However, if you understand that cancer grows in response to lifestyle factors & chronic stress accumulation, you can transform your diagnosis into an opportunity. The opportunity offered as a result of the "message" your body is sending you, is to begin a transformation of all areas of your life that do not truly nourish you, into what is truly nourishing for your body, mind and soul. **This is never easy, but it is your cure.**

To reverse cancer, you must have the courage to face any fears that block you from gaining more clarity about the root cause, and taking action to change your life. For example, taking an honest look at the quality of the relationship(s) in your life, your career, or the environment you live in. You must develop the courage to face the unknown, because that is the nature of change.

Cancer only becomes a serious problem in the late stages of development. Even then, you can still reverse it, it's just harder (much harder) because if pain enters the equation (and it does in late stages of cancer), you then have more sources of stress to deal with. There are some beliefs about cancer that say "cancer is a sign that the body is 'in a healing phase', but this is not true - **don't take cancer lightly.** Do your best to keep your focus on the changes you need to make - **it's the only way healing can occur long-term.**

Remember, you are genetically designed (miraculously) to survive challenges, and more – you are designed to thrive. **Thriving means you live a meaningful life, you are happy about your life, you have the freedom you need to pursue what inspires you, and your body runs optimally and feels great.** Cancer cannot exist in your body if you are truly thriving in life. If you are not thriving, your choices are to begin dreaming about what you want, make goals, and start moving in that direction, or... look for a treatment or a cure, and hope it will somehow solve the problem.

Now you understand why the cure to cancer will never result from a more powerful method to destroy cancer cells – that kind of cure is impossible. A common story I hear from my clients is that the treatments they used before working with me either didn't destroy their cancer successfully, or they were declared cancer-free, only to have cancer reappear a few months later, worse than before. **A war on cancer only perpetuates all the unmet needs in our lives and in humanity, which brought us cancer to begin with.**

The war on cancer has led to and still leads to tremendous loss and suffering, year after year; it keeps the human race stuck in a downward spiral towards "hell". If humanity does not start focusing on the fulfillment of human needs (and this starts with individuals such as you and me), the rate of cancer will likely rise to almost 1 in 1 people.

To reverse cancer, you must believe that you can succeed in the creation of a new reality for yourself which nourishes you from the inside out, and the outside in.

Your life is valuable! If you are alive, it means you have a special contribution that you could make to humanity. The state of our world – the well being of Humanity and Earth – is a reflection of the collective individual choices humanity makes each day. Don't hand your human potential over to the limiting beliefs and values of mainstream society. Don't hand your life over to fear. Open your heart, and dream of a loving future you truly want and deserve, and start taking steps towards it. This is how you take charge of your health, your fate, and your future.

The Truth about cancer that I am sharing with you may not be easy to digest. It means enormous numbers of people have suffered tremendously in a myriad of extreme ways, yet if we had only understood cancer more, things would likely have gone differently. For some people (most, actually), the pain of loss related to cancer is so great that it requires healing through grief-work; effective psyho-emotional processing that leads to a feeling of acceptance of the past - this is not an easy task, however it is up to us to heal ourselves. **To end cancer, we have to do it ourselves** – and that may sound impossible since we've been told for decades that we can't. But we can.

Tumors can exist in a dormant "benign" state or be fast-growing and "aggressive" – definitions that you can now understand, based on what's been presented in this book. The speed of cancer growth differs due to the overall set of stress factors present in each individual's life, which can change moment to moment. If a person undergoes a period of intense, continuous psychological stress, their body would develop more rapidly growing cancer. Another person's overall stress may be relatively low, but still chronic; their body may also grow cancer but at a slower rate. If an individual resolves enough chronic stress, their cancer will stop growing, and if tested, their cancer would be "benign". Most importantly, when a person resolves all stress factors related to the root cause of their cancer, their cancer cells will not only stop growing, but can be cleaned up by the body entirely, and disappear.

Consider the fact that 50% of cancer pap-smear tests which show mild abnormalities, revert to normal within two years without any intervention.[214] Even advanced breast tumours sometimes disappear entirely over six years – without any treatments.[215] These are examples of cancer reversing in people, with no clear healing protocol in place, who likely did not even know the root cause of their cancer. In a 2010 study on breast cancer, half of the 227 women studied with recently diagnosed breast cancer were taught skills to reduce their stress levels; those who completed the stress-reducing program had a 45% reduced risk of breast cancer reoccurring 11 years later.[216] Studies such as this one reveal that we can influence whether cancer grows or not, by addressing psycho-emotional stress factors.

With the right healing protocol in place, cancer can reverse much faster. My program's primary focus was on identifying and resolving all stress-factors that existed prior to their diagnosis, and any current stress-factors, and then changing their life for the better for total resolution. **Most (90%) of my clients had no more symptoms of cancer after only 3 weeks of participating in my reverse cancer residency program, and most had come with either stage 3 or 4 cancer, after traditional and alternative approaches to healing had failed. Most had been given only a few weeks or months to live.**

The Root Cause Work is something that teaches me more and more as my experience with clients grows, hence my ability to help others on their self-healing journey continues to expand.

Should I Worry About Stress?

Fearing stress is counterproductive – rememember it takes substantial periods of chronic stress before cancer builds inside our body. Additionally, recall that on average, a person has cancer for seven years before diagnosis.[217]

However, we should all still take stress seriously: remember to do your best to always grow through life-challenges, if or when they arise. This means being honest about the various kinds of stress that may effect you. In my practice, helping cancer patients heal from within, a common reality I see is that **the life-challenges they have encountered are so difficult to change that they try to "forget about them", which leads to emotional suppression, or denial of what's true.** Suppressing your emotional truth for too long, can not only get you caught in a perpetual reality that does not nourish you – **but it will trigger cancer growth.** When you face your fears and honour what's true, you won't suppress emotional stress; this is how you **grow through the challenges you face,** and get the chance to create a new reality that does nourish you.

Some individuals will need to heal a painful past to prevent or reverse cancer, because resolving the suppressed emotional pain will release the carried stress. Some individuals will need to clean up their diet, start eating real organic, whole food, and drink clean water; some will need to complete a whole-body cleanse or a specific organ cleanse such as for the liver; some will need to resolve current challenges in relationship(s); and some will need to find a new career path, perhaps starting their own business, because it will make life more exciting and meaningful (not based on survival alone). Some will need to simply go on a long vacation, alone (freedom), to find the clarity they need for healing their life.

Positive change starts with a goal – a decision to strive for an improved future. **Once you make a goal, as long as you remain devoted to the process of change, it is only a matter of time before your goal is reached.**

TIP

If you feel overwhelmed by a particular life-challenge or circumstance, start intentionally spending more quality time alone, ideally in nature, so you can hear the messages of your soul. This will also help you build energy to support you through the change process. If you find it difficult to spend time alone, you must work on this. In the meantime, spend time **with someone you feel safe and free with, who believes in you.**

Getting away allows you to regain vital energy because you disconnect from the challenges and responsibilities of life. Turn off your phone for a few hours or even a few days. During that time, practice listening to and trusting your inner voice moment to moment. While alone, you may feel your emotions more; allow yourself to experience whatever feelings arise. Look at your fears. Crying if you need to, and connecting to your truth are some of the highest forms of love that you can give to yourself. **Growing in self-love and self-acceptance is essential for healing.** Only once you've substantially processed your thoughts and feelings, can you move forward with more clarity as to what you need to do with your life to resolve chronic stress and unfulfilled needs.

If you are afraid to be alone or find every reason NOT to go and be alone – then being alone is precisely what you need most. Be courageous! Try doing something different in your life! Face the unknown, and trust!

If we can each become more relaxed in our lives and create

a more balanced life between work and play; if we can build meaning into our lives and feel excited about our future; if we can grow through relationship challenges and reject stagnation; and if we can learn how to trust our inner voice (our Soul); doors will open for us.

If you have self-judgment (negative internal messages or beliefs about yourself or life, that keep you repeating a pattern that isn't good for you or others), learn to notice these thoughts and behaviours, and practice changing them. **Likewise, if you have judgments towards others (learn to understand them and try to see from their perspective; put yourself in their shoes).**

Spontaneous remissions are not anomalies – these can be accomplished consciously. Spiritually speaking, if your belief is "I can," then you have a good chance of taking control of your health and future. If you believe cancer is the result of factors that are out of your control, then you will likely have no choice but hand over your power, health, and maybe your life, to someone else, or a "cure", hoping your cancer can be taken away without any responsibility on your part. **This is a very dangerous spiritual approach to cancer.**

The greatest fear in life may be the fear of death. If cancer cell growth gets triggered in our body because our needs have gone to the wayside, the best response we can make, as soon as possible, is to face this reality head-on, and accept the possibility of dying. This is important so that we don't make all our decisions based on trying to avoid death, rather than on healing ourselves. After we shed fear, we must then decide that we WILL heal, and commit to healing ourselves. We must decide we want to live for a reason that is exciting and meaningful to us, so that it awakens our Soul.

Ironically, an individual must face the potential reality of dying, because only when it is faced can they completely set their focus on positive change (healing). Until then, the fear can keep a strong hold, pulling them down, draining their energy, and sending them in many different directions, fearfully, trying to avoid death. Meanwhile, all the important, positive life changes they need to heal, aren't being made.

We've all been born into a world that needs transformation, positive change, and ultimately, healing. Cultures and societies at large, are not currently able to prepare people to thrive in life. The medical system is usually more focused on prescription drugs than health principles. The school system doesn't teach us life-skills. Our parents can only teach us what they were taught, and can only pass on the personal growth they have made in their own lives. If our parents weren't very healthy or happy, it means we must discover how to create happiness and health ourselves.

Be a leader – heal yourself! Prevent cancer! Go as far as you can each day in your progression towards the fulfilment of your needs. Heal your body by healing every possible aspect of your life. Don't get stuck holding on to "safety" or the "known", sacrificing happiness, freedom, or a purposeful life.

ROOT CAUSE PRACTITIONER TRAINING

Paul, this was an amazing course and I'm so grateful for everything! I've truly learned so much for you and I'm so excited for level 2.

Since finishing the class I've been paying close attention to Free-will and several of the lessons you taught us around love. These teachings helped remind me that I need to always speak up and voice my opinion if something doesn't feel right to me – which I've chosen to do several times in the last week.

These lessons have also improved my leadership skills which again I am most grateful for. Thank you Paul.
-Jill

Hey Paul,

I'm literally blown away with the all information your sharing with regards to our chakra system & the places illness shows up, it's the most fascinating information I've ever heard.

I'm so looking forward to getting into depth of 15 step process tonight. Literally buzzing for it & all of a sudden healing is becoming an amazing journey to be on.
Thanks,
with love Arlene

16

THE CURE IS YOU, AND ALL OF US

The life-circumstances of every individual are unique, and thus the solutions to cancer are as well. Regardless of this fact, there are essential foundation principles of health which apply to us all, for healing cancer.

Here is a list to help you with either the prevention or reversal of cancer:

1. A cancer diagnosis is a message that an aspect of your life is not good for you, so you must change something in order to heal yourself. The thing that is not good for you is either something related to what you are doing, which includes potential beliefs and judgments (most likely without awareness), or it is something that is happening to you that you don't know how to put an end to, or are agreeing to out of fear.

2. Focus on clearing out all the physical sources of stress that may be present in your life – reduce and ideally eliminate processed foods and packaged foods that contain chemicals, refined sugar, additives and "natural flavours", and any food or drink that leads to significant blood glucose surges.

3. Remove pesticides from your diet, and other chemicals, by eating organic whole foods. You may be able to grow your

own garden – and if you decide to do that, you may be surprised at how healing and fulfilling it can be to provide for yourself. Also, there are many lovingly devoted organic farmers out there, who you will likely find if you search for them.

4. Swap toxic body care products, makeup, and cleaning products that contain chemicals, for organic and hand made ones: Find small self-employed entrepreneurs who care about you and our world, and have gone to great lengths to provide hand-made, healthy solutions for these types of products.

5. Focus each day on drinking pure, clean spring water, or filtered and re-mineralized water. You don't need to drink any other liquid than water to be healthy. Teas and freshly squeezed juices, and for some individuals, raw milk can be beneficial, but clean water is still more important. NOTE: many of my clients, prior to working with me, had tried significant juicing protocols only to see their cancer return or never disappear. The reason, which you likely understand now, is that juicing does not address the root cause of cancer.

6. If you have cancer, focus on creating the conditions in your life which will allow your body to deactivate it. **To deactivate cancer, you must diminish your total stress load and unwanted responsibilities, change your lifestyle, and resolve internalized stress.** Be honest with yourself about every aspect of your life, so you can address whatever needs to be addressed.

7. Practice embracing alone time each day – give yourself the space to be free so that you can connect with yourself about all that is going on in your life. Through this connection, you can gain invaluable clarity. The key to beneficial aloneness is creating experiences for yourself in which you

feel free.

8. Realize that your thoughts and emotions have a massive impact on your physical health. **To fulfill your psychological and emotional needs, you must pursue and experience the life that you honestly want.** Thinking positively can be helpful at times, but being completely honest about your reality is crucial. Living in a reality that results in positive thoughts is what heals, and sustains health, longterm.

9. Believe in yourself and love yourself enough to imagine your future the way you'd like to experience it, and then faithfully work towards creating and choosing that reality, surrendering to the process of change, knowing that if you do your part, the rest will take care of itself. **Take the time to write down or draw a picture of what you want your future to look like. NOTE: you cannot control others – this is your journey, and some parts of your journey may need to be walked alone.**

10. **Surround yourself with carefully chosen people, who believe in you and your healing.** Create as much separation as needed from those who do not believe in you, bring you down, or keep you focused on what does not heal you – **keep their fear and negative influence out of your system.** Mismatched relationship values will only drain your energy, and theirs.

Personal Help with Cancer

Book 1 provided you an introductory understanding of the Root Cause of Cancer. Next, Book 2 will focus on the deeper psychological and emotional causes of cancer, and self-healing.

If you are holding this book in your hands, then you are likely

already part of the much-needed paradigm shift required to end cancer and change our world for the better. Thank you.
To help our world continue to grow in consciousness and heal, here are some ways you can help:

11. Apply what you've learned in Book 1. Until you have personal control of your health and life, it's unwise to invest too much time and energy trying to help others. **Put yourself first, with love in your heart.**

12. If you want to develop a professional skillset in the prevention and reversal of cancer, and acquire deep knowledge about advanced principles of self-healing, you can take my Root Cause Practitioner Trainings, Level 1 & 2
    See www.rootcauseinstitute.com

13. If you have cancer and want personal guidance and support in your self-healing process, start with a Root Cause Session, and then complete my Self-Healing Course + Mentorship.

14. If you don't have cancer, but have unresolved life or relationship challenges, and understand that this can lead to cancer, and want to prevent it from developing, you can also hire a Root Cause Practitioner.

Inquire at www.rootcauseinstitute.com

LET'S END CANCER!

REFERENCES

Introduction: The Paradigm Shift

1. https://www.canada.ca/en/public-health/services/chronic-diseases/cancer/canadian-cancer-statistics.html
2. https://www.acc.org/latest-in-cardiology/ten-points-to-remember/2019/02/15/14/39/aha-2019-heart-disease-and-stroke-statistics

Chapter 1: Cancer Is NOT a Disease

3. https://www.cancerresearchuk.org/health-professional/cancer-statistics/risk
4. Servan-Schrieber, MD, PhD. Anticancer: A New Way of Life, Penguin Books. 2017. page 39
5. "Early History of Cancer | American Cancer Society." www.cancer.org, 2018, www.cancer.org/cancer/cancer-basics/history-of-cancer/what-is-cancer.html.
6. Ibid
7. Ibid
8. Ibid
9. Dealing With Cancer Recurrence. 3 May 2019, www.cancer.net/survivorship/dealing-cancer-recurrence.
10. Early History of Cancer | American Cancer Society. www.cancer.org/cancer/cancer-basics/history-of-cancer/what-is-cancer.html.
11. Ibid
12. Ibid
13. Ibid
14. Development of Modern Knowledge about Cancer Causes... www.cancer.org/cancer/cancer-basics/history-of-cancer/modern-knowledge-and-cancer-causes.html.
15. Meng, Xiaolong, et al. "A New Hypothesis for the Cancer Mechanism" Cancer and Metastasis Reviews, vol. 31, no. 1-2, 2011, pp. 247–268., doi:10.1007/s10555-011-9342-8.
16. The Secret History of the War on Cancer, by Devra Lee Davis, BasicBooks, 2007, p.xii.
17. Chopra, Deepak, MD, Michael Murray, ND, and the Metagenics Corp. Exercise Coach Manual, CHEK Institute, pg 23
18. "Cancer Statistics at a Glance – Canadian Cancer Society" www.cancer.ca, 2020, www.cancer.ca/en/cancer-information/cancer-101/cancer-statis-tics-at-a-glance/?region=on

19. Ibid
20. Siegel, Rebecca L., et al. "Cancer Statistics, 2020." CA: A Cancer Journal for Clinicians, vol. 70, no. 1, 2020, pp. 7-30., doi:10.3322/caac.21590
21. "Cancer Statistics for the UK." Cancer Research UK, 5 Mar. 2020 www.cancerresearchuk.org/health-professional/cancer-statistics-for-the-uk
22. Cancer" World Health Organization, World Health Organization, www.who.int/news-room/fact-sheets/detail/cancer
23. Image License ID: 2JTYKGM
24. Haruki, Tomohiro, et al. "Spontaneous Regression of Lung Adenocarcino- ma: Report of a Case." Surgery Today, vol. 40, no. 12, 2010, pp. 1155–1158., doi:10.1007/s00595-009-4195-2.
25. Hardin Jones of National Cancer Institute of Bethesda, Maryland, 1956 Transactions of the NY Academy of Medical Sciences, Vol.6
26. Moritz, Andreas. Cancer Is Not a Disease!: It's a Healing Mechanism: Discover Cancer's Hidden Purpose, Heal Its Root Causes, and Be Healthier than Ever! Ener-Chi Wellness Press, 2017.p11

Chapter 2: Our Bodies Don't Lie

27. McTaggart, Lynne. What Doctors Don't Tell You… The Truth About the Dangers of Modern Medicne, pg. 219-22
28. https://www.ncbi.nlm.nih.gov/pmc/articles/PMC4828728
29. https://www.mossreports.com/when-chemo-kills
30. https://www.lifeextension.com/magazine/1998/1/feature98
31. See Ralph Moss, Questioning Chemotherapy (New York: Equinox Press, 1995)
32. Rabin, Roni Caryn. "You're on the Clock: Doctors Rush Patients out the Door." USA Today, Gannett Satellite Information Network, 20 Apr. 2014, www.usatoday.com/story/news/nation/2014/04/20/doctor-visits-time-crunch-health-care/7822161/)
33. The Body Electric, by Robert O. Becker and Gary Selden, Morrow, 1998, p. 19.
34. Centor RM. To be a great physician, you must understand the whole story. Med Gen Med. 2007;9(1):59.

Chapter 3: There Can Never Be a Cure-The Cure is You

35. World's Smallest Computer Watches You – from Within. 2010, www.nbcnews.com/id/41722559/ns/technology_and_science-tech_and_gadgets/yworlds-smallest-computer-watches-you-within
36. "Canadian Cancer Society." www.cancer.ca, 2018, www.cancer.ca/en/?region=on+80th+birthday

37. Image License ID: 2379846
38. McTaggart, Lynne. The Cancer Handbook: A What Doctors Don't Tell You... www.amazon.com/Cancer-Handbook-What-Doctors-Publication/dp/0953473481. P10 & THREE PERCENT (3%) EFFICACY OF CHEMO-THERAPY TREATMENT ON CANCER CURE, by CARLOS M. GARCÍA, M.D.
39. Permission to use Image: thanks to Devra Davis, Basic Books and www.environmentalhealthtrust.org
40. stanr9 Follow. "Canadian Cancer Statistics 2010 English" LinkedIn Slide-Share, 13 Feb. 2012, www.slideshare.net/stanr9/canadian-cancer-statis-tics-2010-english.p99
41. Ibid.
42. Ibid. p64
43. Personal phone call to the Canadian Cancer Society and National Cancer Institutes, November, 2012
44. "What about Alternative Therapies? – Canadian Cancer Society." www.cancer.ca, 2020, www.cancer.ca/en/cancer-information/diagno-sis-and-treatment/complementary-therapies/choosing-a-complemen-tary-therapy-and-practitioner/what-about-alternative-therapies/?re-gion=mb
45. "Cancer." World Health Organization, World Health Organization, 2020, www.who.int/news-room/fact-sheets/detail/cancer
46. Is the "War on Cancer" Winnable? 40 Years after the... 2020, blogs.scientificamerican.com/observations/is-the-war-on-cancer-winnable-40-years-after-the-unofficial-declaration-the-disease-is-spreading-throughout-the-globe
47. Ibid
48. Permission to use Image: thanks to Devra Davis, Basic Books and www.environmentalhealthtrust.org
49. The Secret History of the War on Cancer, by Devra Lee Davis, BasicBook, 2007, pp. 113-114
50. Tedx Talk: https://youtu.be/vrZef13BSpU, Dr. Deming, Oncologist
51. Ibid
52. How Cancer Works, by Lauren Sompayrac, Jones and Bartlett, 2004, P7
53. Meng, Xiaolong, et al. "A New Hypothesis for the Cancer Mechanism." Cancer and Metastasis Reviews, vol. 31, no. 1-2, 2011, pp. 247-200doi:10.1007/s10555-011-9342-8
54. Sandoiu, Ana. How Does Cancer Evade the Immune System? New... Health News. 2019, www.medicalnewstoday.com/articles/320177
55. Lodi, Dr Thomas. World Cancer Summit, 2011
56. O'hara, Megan, director. The C-Word, 2016, www.rocoeducational.com/the_c_word.
57. The Trophoblast and the Origins of Cancer: One Solution to the Medical Enigma of Our Time, by Nicholas J. Gonzalez and Linda L. Isaacs, New Spring Press, 2009, pp. 45-49.

58. Lipton, Bruce H. The Wisdom of Your Cells: How Your Beliefs Control Your Biology. Sounds True, 2006
59. The Secret History of the War on Cancer, by Devra Lee Davis, Basic-Books, 2007, pp. 8
60. Ibid

Chapter 4: The Body's Survival Mechanisms

61. Human Physiology: an Integrated Approach, by Dee Unglaub Silverthorn et al., Pearson Education, Inc., 2019, p. 6
62. Exercise Coach Manuel, CHEK Institute, pp.22
63. "Homeostasis." Wikipedia, Wikimedia Foundation, 14 May 2020, en.wiki-pedia.org/wiki/Homeostasis
64. Julia Layton "How Fear Works" 13 September 2005. https://science.how-stuffworks.com/life/inside-the-mind/emotions/fear.htm, 7 June 2020
65. "Hypothermia." Wikipedia, Wikimedia Foundation, 21 May 2020, en.wikipedia.org/wiki/Hypothermia.
66. Why Zebras Don't Get Ulcers: the Acclaimed Guide to Stress, Stress-Related Diseases, and Coping, by Robert M. Sapolsky, Henry Holt and Co., 2004, p.11
67. Behrens, E. M. (2019). Cytokines in Cytokine Storm Syndrome. Cytokine Storm Syndrome, 197-207. doi:10.1007/978-3-030-22094-5_12
68. Connealy, Dr Leigh Erin. World Cancer Summit, 2011

Chapter 5: Managing Glucose

69. Written by Editor Updated on 15th January 2019, and Editor. "People with Diabetes Have an Increased Risk of Dehydration as High Blood Glucose Levels Lead to Decreased Hydration in the Body."Diabetes,11 Mar.2020, www.diabetes.co.uk/dehydration-and-diabetes.html
70. Sugar Blues, by William Dufty, Warner, 1993, pp. 149–152.
71. Ibid. pg 137
72. Calder, Sherry. "New Diabetes Rates Released with Urgent Plea for Gorvernments to Implement National Diabetes Strategy." Diabetes-CanadaWebsite, 2019, www.diabetes.ca/media-room/press-releases/new-diabetes-rates-released-with-urgent-plea-for-governments-to-implement-national-diabetes-strategy
73. https://www.diabetes.co.uk/stress-and-blood-glucose-levels.html, Roberts, Ff. "Stress and the General Adaptation Syndrome." Bmj, vol.2 no. 4670, 1950, pp. 104–105., doi:10.1136/bmj.2.4670.104-a. 2020, www.diabetes.co.uk/dehydration-and-diabetes.html

Chapter 6: Fight or Flight

74. Why Zebras Don't Get Ulcers: the Acclaimed Guide to Stress, Stress-Related Diseases, and Coping, by Robert M. Sapolsky, Henry Holt and Co., 2004, p.30-32
75. Adrenal Fatigue: the 21st Century Stress Syndrome, by James L. Wilson,Smart Publications, 2017, p. 6
76. Ibid
77. Why Zebras Don't Get Ulcers: the Acclaimed Guide to Stress, Stress-Related Diseases, and Coping, by Robert M. Sapolsky, Henry Holt and Co., 200% P.122
78. The Relationship of Stress to Hypoglycemia and Alcoholism, Kathryn Carron Poulos, C. Jean & Donald Stoddard, International Institute of Natural Health Sciences, 1979, pg 10-11, The Emergency Function of the Adrenal Medulla in Pain and the Major Emotions, American Journal of Physiology,33:356, 1914. Wisdom of the Body, New York. WW Norton, 1939
79. Ibid
80. Ibid
81. Ibid
82. Why Zebras Don't Get Ulcers: the Acclaimed Guide to Stress, Stress-Related Discases, and Coping, by Robert M. Sapolsky, Henry Holt and Co.,2004, p. 34
83. Vibrational Medicine: the #1 Handbook of Subtle-Energy Therapies, by Richard Gerber, Bear & Co., 2001, p. 165
84. Ibid
85. Why Zebras Don't Get Ulcers: the Acclaimed Guide to Stress,Stress-Related Discases, and Coping, by Robert M. Sapolsky, Henry Holt and Co.,2004, p. 6-7
86. Tarkan, Laurie. Cancer Patients Feel Less Distress after Massage Therapy... 2013, www.foxnews.com/health/cancer-patients-feel-less-distress-after-massage-therapy-study-finds

Chapter 7: Glucose Feeds Cancer Cells

87. Sherman, E. (2019, February 21). U.S. Health Care Costs Skyrocketed to $3.65 Trillion in 2018. Retrieved July 06, 2020, from https://fortune.com/2019/02/21/us-health-care-costs-2
88. Kvly. "The World's Healthiest Countries, Ranked." News, 2019, www.valleynewslive.com/content/news/The-worlds-healthiest-countries-ranked-506358531.html
89. Ritchie, Hannah. "How Many People in the World Die from Cancer?" Our World in Data, 2018, ourworldindata.org/how-many-people-in-the-

world-die-from-cancer
90. "Early History of Cancer | American Cancer Society." www.cancer.org, 2018, www.cancer.org/cancer/cancer-basics/history-of-cancer/what-is-cancer.html
91. The Secret History of the War on Cancer, by Devra Lee Davis, Basic-Books, 2007, p.214
92. The Emperor of All Maladies: a Biography of Cancer, by Siddhartha-Mukherjee, Gale, Cengage Learning, 2012, pp. 87–91
93. Chang, Louise. "Side-Effects of Radiation Therapy for Cancer Treatment." www.webmd.com, 2018, www.webmd.com/cancer/what-to-expect-from-radiation-therapy
94. "Managing the Lingering Side Effects of Cancer Treatment." Mayo Clinic. February 19, 2019. Accessed July 12, 2020. https://www.mayoclinic.org/diseases-conditions/cancer/in-depth/cancer-survivor/art-20045524?f-bclid=IwAR23AcqgWjBd18pu3pw02P_Kq6MVeX-BaUyWVOGltfS6U-WrUYX5wP8CDpp2A
95. Chemo Side-Effects Info at Susan G. Komen, (n.d.). Retrieved July 12,2020, from https://ww5.komen.org/BreastCancer/LongTermSideEf-fectsof-Chemotherapy.html?fbclid=IwARIAAmLfzOLHuHu5n4Y43b-8Bus8zsjGYizv_lx4z7WWqxQHnGcFBOm7vs5E
96. "Managing the Lingering Side Effects of Cancer Treatment?" February 19, 2019. Accessed July 12, 2020. https://www.mayoclinic.org/diseas-es-conditions/cancer/in-depth/cancer-survivor/art-20045524?fbclid=I-WARO_FjKAyFS9p7i87-iM-mcWGCbG9_ltl114D6cCFy3NqMiUehWxC0d-PmTM.
97. Kingsley, Patrick. Cancer Teleseminar, 2011"Managing the Lingering Side Effects of Cancer Treatment." Mayo Clinic. February 19, 2019. Accessed July 12, 2020. https://www.mayoclinic.org/diseases-conditions/cancer/in-depth/cancer-survivor/art-20045524?fbclid=IwAR23AcqgWjBd-18pu3pw02P_Kq6MVeXBaUywVOGlf$6UWrUYX5wP8CDpp2A
98. Lodi, Dr Thomas. World Cancer Summit. 2011
99. "Oxygen Therapies." What Doctors Don't Tell You, 2000, www.wddty.com/oxygen-therapies.html
100. Human Physiology: an Integrated Approach, by Dee Unglaub Silverthorn et al., Pearson Education, Inc., 2019, p. 359.
101. ScienceBlog.com. "Does Sugar Feed Cancer?" ScienceBlog.com, 17 Aug.2009, scienceblog.com/24162/does-sugar-feed-cancer
102. Ibid
103. Beating Cancer with Nutrition: Harnessing the Incredible Healing Power of Nature and Science.., by Patrick Quillin and Noreen Quillin, Nutrition Times Press, 2005, p. 121
104. Connealy, DR Leigh Erin. World Cancer Summit, 2011
105. How Cancer Works, by Lauren Sompayrac, Jones and Bartlett, 2004, p.7
106. Moynihan, Timothy. "Heart Cancer: Is There Such a Thing? – Mayo Clinic"

Mayoclinic.org, 2019, www.mayoclinic.org/heart-cancer/expert-answers/faq-20058130

Chapter 8: 100 Pounds of Poison

107. How to Eat, Move and Be Healthy: Your Personalized 4-Step Guide to Looking and Feeling Great from the inside Out, by Paul Chek, C.H.E.K. Institute, 2018, p. 76. Halstead, Bruce W., et al. "Poison." Encyclopædia Britannica, Encyclopædia Britannica, Inc., 14 May 2019, www.britannica.com/science/poison-biochemistry
108. Bennett JM, Rodrigues IM, Klein LC. Effects of caffeine and stress on biomarkers of cardiovascular disease in healthy men and women with a family history of hypertension. Stress Health. 2013;29(5):401-9. doi:10.1002/smi.2486
109. Sugar Blues, by William Dufty, Warner, 1993, pp. 22-23.
110. Molecules of Emotion, by Candace B. Ph. D. Pert, Scribner, 1997, p. 298.
111. Briffa, John. "How Cutting out Sugar Can Help Earache | Daily Mail Online." www.dailymail.co.uk,www.dailymail.co.uk/health/article-28379/How-cutting-sugar-help-earache.html. Sanchez, Albert, et al. "Role of Sugars in Human Neutrophilic Phagocytosis." The American Journal of Clinical Nutrition, vol. 26, no. 11, 1973, pp. 1180-1184., doi:10.1093/ajcn/26.11.1180
112. "How Many Drinks Does The Coca-Cola Company Sell Worldwide Each Day?: Frequently Asked Questions: Coca-Cola NG" Coca, 2020, www.coca-cola.com.ng/our-company/faqs/how-many-cans-of-coca-cola-are-sold-worldwide-in-a-day
113. Facts about Sweeteners and Sugar Substitutes, www.sugar-and-sweetener-guide.com
114. Powderley, Kathleen. "One in Three Canadians Is Living with Diabetes or Prediabetes, Yet Knowledge of Risk and Complications of Disease Remains Low." DiabetesCanadaWebsite, 2019, www.diabetes.ca/media-room/press-releases/one-in-three-canadians-is-living-with-diabetes-or-prediabetes,-yet-knowledge-of-risk-and-complication
115. Chopra, Deepak, MD, Michael Murray, ND, and the Metagenics Corp. Exercise Coach Manual, CHEK Institute, pg 23
116. Sugar Blues, by William Dufty, Warner, 1993, pp. 149-152
117. P, Surat. "PH in the Human Body." News, 24 Aug. 2018, www.news-medical.net/health/pH-in-the-Human-Body.aspx
118. Sugar Blues, by William Dufty, Warner, 1993, pp. 137.
119. https://www.unisa.edu.au/media-centre/Releases/2021/caffeine-cuts-close-to-the-bon--when-it-comes-to-osteoporosis/
120. https://www.medicalnewstoday.com/articles/how-common-is-osteoporosis#by-country

Chapter 9: Poison Disguised

121. ScienceBlog.com. "Does Sugar Feed Cancer?" ScienceBlog.com, 17 Aug. 2009, scienceblog.com/24162/does-sugar-feed-cancer
122. Liu, H., et al. "Fructose Induces Transketolase Flux to Promote Pancreatic Cancer Growth." Cancer Research, vol. 70, no. 15, 2010, pp. 6368–6376.,doi:10.1158/0008-5472.can-09-4615
123. How to Eat, Move and Be Healthy: Your Personalized 4-Step Guide to Looking and Feeling Great from the inside Out, by Paul Chek, C.H.E.K. Institute, 2018, p. 58
124. https://www.britannica.com/technology/pasteurization
125. Milk the Deadly Poison, by CohenRobert, Argus, 1998, p. 211
126. Nourishing Traditions: the Cookbook That Challenges Politically Correct Nutrition and the Diet Dictocrats, by Sally Fallon et al., NewTrendsPublishing, Inc., 2005, pp. 30-35., https://www.breastfeedingnetwork.org.uk/cholesterol
127. Holistic Lifestyle Coaching, Level 1, Paul Chek, C.H.E.K. Institute, 2012
128. Getoff, David. Personal phone conversation. 2012
129. Bricker, A., Douglass, A., Garcia, D. K., Hayes, R., Imhoff, D., Kimbrell,A., & Naylor, G. (n.d.). Issues: | GE Foods. Retrieved June 26, 2020,from https://www.centerforfoodsafety.org/issues/311/ge-foods/ge-food-and-your-health
130. Gross and Microscopic Anatomy of the Small Intestine, www.vivo.colostate.edu/hbooks/pathphys/digestion/smallgut/anatomy.html
131. Hare, Christian O, and Name *. "Food Intolerance May Be Making You Tired and Fat!" Thrive, 10 Apr. 2019, www.thrivehealth.fitness/food-intolerance-may-be-making-you-tired-and-fat/.
132. "Gluten: What You Don't Know Might Kill You" Dr. Mark Hyman, 25 Nov. 2019, drhyman.com/blog/2011/03/17/gluten-what-you-dont-know-might-kill-you
133. No Wheat, No Problem!: Easy Recipes & Strategies for Living Gluten Free, by Corrie Ann Materie, DCM Publications, 2003, pp. 12–13
134. Personal Conversation with Paul Chek. CHEK Institute, 2011

Chapter 10: Garbage In, Garbage Out

135. The Politics of Cancer Revisited, by Samuel S. Epstein and P. Mineau, East Ridge Press, 1998, pp. 117-180
136. tsmith on July 13, 2010. "Tsmith." ScienceBlogs, 2010, scienceblogs.com/aetiology/2010/07/13/the-importance-of-gut-flora
137. Chopra, Deepak. What Is the True Nature of Reality?, 1991, ascen-sion-research.org/reality.html.
138. ibid

139. Farlow, Christine Hoza. Food Additives: a Shopper's Guide to Whats Safe & What's Not. KISS for Health Pub., 2013

140. Beating the Food Giants, by Paul A. Stitt, Natural Press, 1993, p.127

141. Bricker, A., Douglass, A., Garcia, D. K., Hayes, R., Imhoff, D., Kimbrell,A., & Naylor, G. (n.d.). Isues: | GE Foods. Retrieved June 26, 2020,from https://www.centerforfoodsafety.org/issues/311/ge-foods/ge-food-and-your-health

142. www.echovallygrassfedbeef.com, www.dobsonfarm.com, www.mcsmith-sorganicfarm.com, beyondfactoryfarming.org, www.stopfactoryfarms.org. Personal experience raising my own animals.

143. Center for Food Safety and Applied Nutrition. "Generally Recognized as Safe (GRAS)" Accessed June 09, 2020. https://www.fda.gov/food/food-ingredients-packaging/generally-recognized-as-safe-gras

144. Zeitgeist: Moving Forward--Trilogy. Directed by Peter Joseph. Sideways Film, 2010

145. Bailor, Jonathan. The Smarter Science of Slim: What the Actual Experts Have Proven about Weight Loss, Health, and Fitness. New York: Aavia Publishing, 2012. 157

146. Schmidt, C. W. (1998). Childhood cancer: A growing problem. Environmental Health Perspectives, 106(1). doi:10.1289/ehp.98106a18

147. The Politics of Cancer Revisited, by Samuel S. Epstein and P. Mineau, East Ridge Press, 1998, pp. 531

148. Ibid. pg. 116

149. How to Eat, Move and Be Healthy: Your Personalized 4-Step Guide to Looking and Feeling Great from the inside Out, by Paul Chek, C.H.E.K. Institute, 2018. Audio series: Are we the biggest guinea pigs in the biggest scientific experiment?

150. The Politics of Cancer Revisited, by Samuel S. Epstein and P. Mineau, East Ridge Press, 1998, pp. 39

151. How to Eat, Move and Be Healthy: Your Personalized 4-Step Guide to Looking and Feeling Great from the inside Out, by Paul Chek, C.H.E.K. Institute, 2018.p58

152. Ibid pg 59

153. "EWG Skin Deep° Cosmetics Database." EWG. Accessed June 09, 2020. https://www.ewg.org/skindeep

154. How to Eat, Move and Be Healthy: Your Personalized 4-Step Guide to Looking and Feeling Great from the inside Out, by Paul Chek, C.H.E.K. Institute, 2018.p59

155. "Sweet Misery: A Poisoned World - Top Documentary Films." Accessed June 9, 2020. https://topdocumentaryfilms.com/sweet-misery-a-poisoned-world

156. Ibid, Spartame: The Dangers and Side Effects (Part 1 of 3). Directed by Mercola. Accessed 2020. https://www.youtube.com/watch?v=Jk-SladbM-SPo&feature=youtu.be.

157. Ibid
158. Calton, Mira, and Jayson Calton. Rebuild Your Bones: The 12-week Osteoporosis Protocol. New York: Rodale Books, 2019
159. Nakanishi, Yuko, Koichi Tsuneyama, Makoto Fujimoto, Thucydides L. Salunga, Kazuhiro Nomoto, Jun-Ling An, Yasuo Takano, Seiichi Iizuka, Mitsunobu Nagata, Wataru Suzuki, Tsutomu Shimada, Masaki Aburada, Masayuki Nakano, Carlo Selmi, and M. Eric Gershwin. "Monosodium Glutamate (MSG): A Villain and Promoter of Liver Inflammation and Dysplasia." Journal of Autoimmunity 30, no. 1-2 (2008): 42-50. doi:10.1016/j.jaut.2007.11.016

Chapter 11: Being Stuck in Stress Can Trigger Cancer

160. B Stress Quotes, Relaxation Sayings, Quotations about Tension. Accessed June 09, 2020. http://www.quotegarden.com/stress.html.
161. Nerburn, Kent (edited By). The Wisdom of the Native Americans. New York, NY: MJF Books, 2009.
162. Wharton, Charles Heizer. Metabolic Man: Ten Thousand Years from Eden. Orlando, FL: Winmark Pub., 2001. P.xxiii
163. Price, Weston Andrew. Nutrition and Physical Degeneration. Lemon Grove, CA: Price-Pottenger, 2016.
164. Ibid
165. Nerburn, Kent (edited By). The Wisdom of the Native Americans. New York, NY: MJF Books, 2009.
166. Wilson, Edward O. The Future of Life. Random House, 2003. 99-100.
167. Ibid. pg 25
168. Wharton, Charles Heizer. Metabolic Man: Ten Thousand Years from Eden. Orlando, FL: Winmark Pub., 2001. P.40
169. Ibid
170. Personal Conversation with Paul Chek. Laura, Derrick, Kitty, Josh, Danielle, Jason Sandeman, Jenn, Karen, Alison Golden, Katy, Mark Sisson, Kishore, Nicky Spur, Tony, Brian Kozmo, Ely, Dawn, Celeste, Cathy, Tamara, Joe Brancaleone, Tim, Bea Binag, Ian, Wes, Marty, Fred Smith, Bobby Fernandez, Michael, Bryan, and Kelda. "The Characteristics of Hunter-Gatherer Fitness." Mark's Daily Apple. November 14, 2013. Accessed June 09, 2020. https://www.marksdailyapple.com/the-characteristics-of-hunter-gatherer-fitness
171. 168 Wharton, Charles Heizer. Metabolic Man: Ten Thousand Years from Eden. Orlando, FL: Winmark Pub., 2001. P.40
172. Comparing more and less developed countries. (2018, September 12) Retrieved July 01, 2020, from https://www.wcrf.org/dietandcancer/cancer-trends/comparing-more-and-less-developed-countries
173. Goldstein, Carly M., Richard Josephson, Susan Xie, and Joel W. Hughes.

"Current Perspectives on the Use of Meditation to Reduce Blood Pressure" International Journal of Hypertension 2012 (2012): 1-11. doi:10.1155/2012/578397

174. Sinha, Shashankshekhar, Ajaykumar Jain, Sanjay Tyagi, Sk Gupta, and Aartisood Mahajan. "Effect of 6 Months of Meditation on Blood Sugar,Glycosylated Hemoglobin, and Insulin Levels in Patients of Coronary Artery Disease." International Journal of Yoga 11, no. 2 (2018): 122. doi:10.4103/ijoy.ijoy_30_17

175. Ferris, Emma. "The Power Of Your Breath." The Breath Effect. April 22, 2020. Accessed July 01, 2020. https://www.thebreatheffect.com/the-power-of-your-breath

176. "How Common Is Divorce and What Are the Reasons?" How Common Is Divorce and What Are the Reasons? | Your Divorce Questions. Accessed June 09, 2020. https://yourdivorcequestions.org/how-common-is-divorce

177. "How Stress Affects Cancer Risk | MD Anderson Cancer Center." Accessed June 9, 2020. https://www.mdanderson.org/publications/focused-on-health/how-stress-affects-cancer-risk.h21-1589046.html

178. "Stress and the Sensitive Gut - Harvard Health." Accessed June 9, 2020. https://www.health.harvard.edu/newsletter_article/stress-and-the-sensitive-gut. "Stress Effects on the Body." Accessed June 9, 2020. https://www.apa.org/helpcenter/stress-body

Chapter 12: Cancer's Location in the Body is Not Random

179. Quillin, Patrick, and Noreen Quillin. Beating Cancer with Nutrition: Harnessing the Incredible Healing Power of Nature and Science ... Carlsbad,CA: Nutrition Times Press, 2005. 324. The Politics of Cancer Revisited, by Samuel S. Epstein and P. Mineau, East Ridge Press, 1998, pp. 3-4,20

180. Cancer. (n.d.). Retrieved July 08, 2020, from https://www.who.int/newsroom/fact-sheets/detail/cancer

181. The Politics of Cancer Revisited, by Samuel S. Epstein and P. Mineau, East Ridge Press, 1998, pp. 28

182. "Sweet Misery: A Poisoned World - Top Documentary Films." Accessed June 9, 2020. https://topdocumentaryfilms.com/sweet-misery-a-poisoned-world

183. Alavanja, Michael C. R., and Matthew R. Bonner. "Occupational Pesticide Exposures and Cancer Risk: A Review." Journal of Toxicology and Environmental Health, Part B 15, no. 4 (2012): 238-63. doi:10.1080/10937404.2012.632358

184. https://pubmed.ncbi.nlm.nih.gov/3912986/, (Scand J Work Environ Health. 1985 Dec;11(6):397-407. doi: 10.5271/sjweh.2208.)

185. Human Physiology: an Integrated Approach, by Dee Unglaub Silverthorn et al., Pearson Education, Inc., 2019, p. 328 Why Zebras Don't Get Ulcers: the Acclaimed Guide to Stress, Stress-Related Diseases, and Coping, by Robert M.Sapolsky, Henry Holt and Co., 2004, p. 23,188

186. Ibid

187. The Politics of Cancer Revisited, by Samuel S. Epstein and P. Mineau, East Ridge Press, 1998, pp.694-95. Why Zebras Don't Get Ulcers: the Acclaimed Guide to Stress, Stress-Related Diseases, and Coping, by Robert M. Sapolsky,Henry Holt and Co., 2004, p. 188. Servan-Schreiber, David. Anticancer: A New Way of Life. NY, NY: Penguin Books, 2017. 35-36. The Editors of Encyclopaedia Britannica. "Inflammation." Encyclopædia Britannica. September 13, 2019. Accessed June 09, 2020. https://www.britannica.com/science/inflammation

188. "Inflammation Linked to Cancer, but Lifestyle Changes May Help" Cancer Treatment Centers of America. January 22, 2020. Accessed June 09,2020. https://www.cancercenter.com/community/blog/2018/08/inflammation-linked-to-cancer-but-lifestyle-changes-may-help

189. Servan-Schreiber, David. Anticancer: A New Way of Life. NY, NY: Penguin Books, 2017. 35-36. "Ihe Stress Response to Injury and Infection.."- Medscape. December 01, 2000. Accessed June 09, 2020. http://www.medscape.com/viewarticle/407543

190. Ke, Po-Yuan, and Steve S.-L. Chen. "Hepatitis C Virus and Cellular Stress Response: Implications to Molecular Pathogenesis of Liver Diseases." Viruses 4, no. 10 (2012): 2251-290. doi:10.3390/v4102251

191. "HPV and Cancer." National Cancer Institute. Accessed June 09, 2020. http://www.cancer.gov/cancertopics/factsheet/risk/HPV

192. Dale, Cyndi, and Richard Wehrman. The Subtle Body: An Encyclopedia of Your Energetic Anatomy. Boulder, CO: Sounds True, 2009. 225

193. Ibid

194. Truman, Karol Kuhn. "Feelings Buried Alive Never Die-- ". Phoenix, AZ:Olympus Distributing, 2015

195. Gonzalez, Nicholas J., and Linda L. Isaacs. The Trophoblast and the Origins of Cancer: One Solution to the Medical Enigma of Our Time. New York,NY: New Spring Press, 2009. 43-49

Chapter 13: Cancer cannot be the result of a cellular error

196. How to Eat, Move and Be Healthy: Your Personalized 4-Step Guide to Looking and Feeling Great from the inside Out, by Paul Chek, C.H.E.K. Institute, 2018.preface p3

197. DeCava, Judith A. The Real Truth about Vitamins and Anti-oxidants, Fort Collins, CO: Selene River Press, 2006. 7

198. Chopra, Deepak. What Is the True Nature of Reality? Accessed June

09.2020. http://ascension-research.org/reality.html.

199. Meng, Xiaolong, Jie Zhong, Shuying Liu, Mollianne Murray, and Ana M.Gonzalez-Angulo. "A New Hypothesis for the Cancer Mechanism." Cancer and Metastasis Reviews 31, no, 1-2 (2011): 247-68. doi:10.1007/s10555-011-9342-8

200. Ibid

201. Karp, Gerald, and Nancy L. Pruitt. Cell and Molecular Biology. Concepts and Experiments. Hoboken, NJ: John Wiley & Sons, 2008. 589-90

202. "Lightning Strike Probabilities." Lightning Strike Probabilities - National Lightning Safety Institute. Accessed June 09, 2020. http://lightningsafety.com/nlsi_pls/probability.html

203. "What Are Your Odds Of Winning the Lottery?" Wonderopolis. Accessed June 09, 2020. https://www.wonderopolis.org/wonder/what-are-your-odds-of-winning-the-lottery

204. Haltiwanger, John. "If You're Afraid Of Flying, The Odds Of A Plane Crash Will Reassure You" Elite Daily. October 02, 2019. Accessed June 09,2020. https://www.elitedaily.com/news/world/people-terrified-plane-crashes-even-though-rare/977885

205. Karp, Gerald, and Nancy L. Pruitt. Cell and Molecular Biology. Concepts and Experiments. Hoboken, NJ: John Wiley & Sons, 2008. 94

206. Human Physiology: an Integrated Approach, by Dee Unglaub Silverthorn et al., Pearson Education, Inc., 2019, p. 79-81

Chapter 14: Our Body Facilitates Cancer Cell Growth

207. Gonzalez, Nicholas J., and Linda L. Isaacs. The Trophoblast and the Origins of Cancer: One Solution to the Medical Enigma of Our Time. New York,NY: New Spring Press, 2009. 43-49

208. Ibid

209. Ibid

210. Ibid

211. Ibid

212. Ibid

213. Murray, Michael, and Bruce Lessey. "Embryo Implantation andTumor Metastasis: Common Pathways of Invasion and Angiogenesis." Seminars in Reproductive Medicine 17, no. 03 (1999): 275-90. doi:10.1055/s-2007-1016235

Chapter 15: The cure is you, and all of us

214. BMJ, 1988; 297: 18-21 McTaggart, Lynne. The Cancer Handbook. Place of Publication Not Identified: What Doctors Don't Tell You, 2000. 48

215. Archives of Internal Medicine, 2008; 168: 2311-2316. McTaggart, Lynne. The Cancer Handbook. Place of Publication Not Identified: WhatDoctors Don't Tell You, 2000. 48

216. Clinical Cancer Research, 2010; doi: 10.1158/1078-0432.CCR-10-0278. McTaggart, Lynne. The Cancer Handbook. Place of Publication Not Identified: What Doctors Don't Tell You, 2000. 48

217. Gordon, Gary. World Cancer Summit, 2011. Gordonresearch.com. Accessed June 09, 2020. http://www.Gordonresearch.comww